AF344267

Prepare for the MRCPsych CASC Exam

Nadiya Sivaswamy

Prepare for the MRCPsych CASC Exam

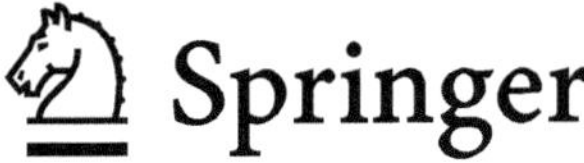 Springer

Nadiya Sivaswamy
Aberdeen, UK

ISBN 978-3-031-31018-8   ISBN 978-3-031-31019-5   (eBook)
https://doi.org/10.1007/978-3-031-31019-5

This Springer imprint is published by the registered company Springer Nature Switzerland AG
The registered company address is: Gewerbestrasse 11, 6330 Cham, Switzerland

To my parents, my father Sivaswamy and mother Kalaimani. For your love, sacrifice and unwavering support.

To my family Kruba, Thushin and Nyra for all your love.

Preface

This book is a product of my own preparation for the CASC exam. There were several resources available for the CASC; however, there was no one resource that would form the scaffold of my CASC preparation. This book is intended to be a one-stop shop for commonly encountered clinical assessments that could feature in the CASC exam. The book features over a 100 high-yield clinical scenarios. This book distinguishes itself from other resources by emphasising a structured approach in each scenario. This maximises candidates' ability to complete every scenario in 7 min as per the RCPSYCH CASC blueprint. Key areas for a particular scenario are highlighted under the station-specific points that allows candidates to understand the salient aspects for a station. This book is intended to be an up-to-date and comprehensive resource for MRCPsych CASC preparation. Candidates are encouraged to use this book in tandem with CASC PREPARE COURSE sessions for maximum benefit. However whether used along with the CASC PREPARE COURSE one to one tutoring and mock exam or in its own, I anticipate that this book will be a valuable addition to your CASC preparation arsenal.

The RCPSYCH CASC exam comprises 16 stations with 7 min for candidates to complete every station. The reading time is 4 min for the first set of eight stations and 90 s for the next set of eight stations. The stations focus on history, management and examination. In addition, stations can also evaluate other areas like capacity assessment and risk assessment. Communication skills are tested in every station in the CASC. Candidates may refer to the RCPSYCH website for latest information about the CASC exam.

Contents

General Adult Psychiatry 1

Old-Age Psychiatry 35

Child and Adolescent Psychiatry and Learning Disability 49

Substance and Alcohol Misuse 63

Liaison Psychiatry 77

Eating Disorders 91

Forensic Psychiatry 99

Psychotherapy 117

Perinatal Psychiatry 131

Explanations 143

Capacity Assessment 157

Examination 167

Index 181

About the Author

Nadiya Sivaswamy I am a psychiatrist and completed my core psychiatry training in the United Kingdom. I successfully qualified for the MRCPsych after passing the CASC with 15 out of 16 stations. I subsequently passed my higher trainee interview and continue working in the National Health Service (NHS) in the United Kingdom as a registrar. I have a special interest in teaching and have a postgraduate certificate in medical education. I am founder of the CASC PREPARE COURSE providing high-quality, personalised one-to-one tutoring, mock exams and ST4 interview sessions. Through CASC PREPARE, we have mentored numerous candidates to successfully navigate and pass their MRCPsych CASC exam. We have excellent testimonials on our website www.cascprepare.com to attest to the high quality of our services.

General Adult Psychiatry

Post-traumatic Stress Disorder

Scenario

42-year-old Thomas Irvine has been referred by the GP since he has been having some issues with his colleagues at work.

Task

Take a history and explore psychopathology.

Approach

Hello, I am Dr. _____. I am a psychiatrist. I understand you have been having some difficulties at work. I am sorry to hear that. Please could you tell me more?

History of Presenting Complaint
- May I ask what difficulties you are experiencing at work?
- When did this all start?
- What was happening in your life at that time [1]?
- The actor will reveal a traumatic event, for example a road traffic accident or being the victim of a robbery.

All names and scenarios mentioned in this book are fictitious. Any resemblance to actual individuals or backgrounds is entirely conincidental.

© The Author(s), under exclusive license to Springer Nature Switzerland AG 2023
N. Sivaswamy, *Prepare for the MRCPsych CASC Exam*,
https://doi.org/10.1007/978-3-031-31019-5_1

Elicit Details of the Traumatic Event
- How serious was it?
- Were you injured?
- Was anybody else injured?
- Any ongoing stressors associated with the event—court case, legal proceedings or compensation claims?

Elicit the Core Symptoms of Post-traumatic Stress Disorder

Hyperarousal
- Persistent anxiety about things going wrong
- Irritability
- Decreased concentration
- Insomnia
- Increased startle response

Re-experiencing
- Vivid flashbacks
- Nightmares of the event

Avoidance of Reminders of the Event
- Place
- People
- Activities

Emotional numbness [2]

Impact and Coping

This sounds really difficult for you. How has this impacted on your

- Relationships
- Work

With all this going on, how have you been coping?

- May I ask if you take alcohol in excess?
- May I ask if you take any recreational drugs?

Psychiatric History

Have you seen a psychiatrist in the past?

Family History

Anyone in the family with any mental or physical health issues?

Medication and Compliance

Do you take any regular medication?

Do you take the medication as prescribed?

Brief Mental State Examination

Ask about mood, sleep, appetite, anhedonia, generalised anxiety, and auditory and visual hallucinations.

Risk Assessment

Suicidal thoughts or plans, thoughts of harming others and deliberate self-harm [1]

Station-Specific Points

- Anticipate that the actor will have difficulty speaking about the traumatic event.
- Be empathic and reassuring in your approach.

Obsessive Compulsive Disorder

Scenario

28-year-old Elizabeth Shaw delivered a baby 6 weeks ago. She has seen her GP today as she is struggling with worrisome thoughts regarding the baby. The GP has referred her to psychiatry for an outpatient appointment.

Task

Take a history to arrive at a provisional diagnosis.

Approach

Hello, I am Dr. ____. I am a psychiatrist. I understand you have been having some difficulties. I am sorry to hear that. Please could you tell me more?

History of Presenting Complaint

- When did all this first start?
- What was happening in your life at that time?
- Has anything like this happened before?
- Are there any triggers that make you think this way?
- Is there anything that makes these thoughts better or worse?
- Do you have any other children?
- How was your pregnancy with this child?
- How is your relationship with your partner [1]?

Elicit the Core Symptoms of Obsessive Compulsive Disorder

Obsessions

- Do you get any unpleasant thoughts, images or recurrent impulses?
- How often do you get these thoughts?
- How long do these thoughts last when they do occur?
- Are they your own thoughts or are they put into your head by an external force?
- How do you feel when you get these thoughts—do these thoughts make you anxious?
- Do you try to stop these thoughts?
- What happens when you do try to stop these thoughts?
- What do you do when you get these thoughts?

Compulsions

- Do you find yourself doing certain things over and over again?
- Does this have to be a certain number of times?
- How much time do you spend in a day doing this?
- Do you do other things like checking, counting and touching objects?
- What happens when you do not do these things?
- How do you feel after you do this?
- May I ask how many hours in a day you spend doing these things [3]?

Impact and Coping

This sounds really difficult for you. How has this impacted on your

- Relationships
- Work
- Ability to care for the baby

  With all this going on, how have you been coping?

- May I ask if you take alcohol in excess?
- May I ask if you take any recreational drugs?

Psychiatric History

Have you seen a psychiatrist in the past?

Family History

Anyone in the family with any mental or physical health issues?

Medication and Compliance

Do you take any regular medication?

    Do you take the medication as prescribed?

Brief Mental State Examination

Ask about mood, sleep, appetite, anhedonia, generalised anxiety, and auditory and visual hallucinations.

Risk Assessment

- Suicidal thoughts or plans, thoughts of harming others and deliberate self-harm
- Do you have any thoughts of washing the baby?
- Do you neglect the baby due to your rituals [1]?

Station-Specific Points

- Risk assessment to include potential harm to the child including thoughts of washing baby and neglecting baby

---

Gender Dysphoria

Scenario

32-year-old Simon Wilson has been referred to psychiatric services by the GP as he wishes to undergo gender reassignment surgery.

Task

Take a history and answer any questions about the process of gender reassignment.

Approach

Hello, I am Dr. _____. I am a psychiatrist. I understand you have been referred by the GP as you have decided to have gender reassignment. May I ask how I can address you? May I ask you a few questions?

History of Presenting Complaint

- May I ask how long you have felt this sense of discomfort with your gender?
- What have you done to experience membership of the opposite gender?
- Have you changed your name officially?
- Have you removed your facial/body hair?
- Cross dressing—may I ask if this was associated with sexual arousal?
- Have you been living full time or part time as a member of the opposite gender?

Childhood/Social History
- How would you describe your childhood?
- May I ask if you have had any difficult experiences like abuse?
- Did you cross dress in clothes of the opposite gender?
- Did you have a preference of toys or games?
- May I ask what your experience of puberty was like?

Relationships
- Are you in a relationship at present?
- May I ask if your partner is male or female?
- How would you describe your sexual orientation?

Impact and Coping
This sounds really difficult for you. How has this impacted?

- Relationships
- Work
- Psychologically

Explain the Process of Gender Reassignment
- High-dose hormonal therapy: We will monitor for side effects like changes in liver function, increased blood pressure, increased blood sugar, and formation of blood clots.
- Surgery—orchidectomy/penectomy.
- Inform that the surgery is irreversible.
- May I ask how certain you are that you would like to change your gender?
- Is there a chance once you begin treatment you may change your mind?
- With your permission, I will refer to the gender reassignment clinic.
- You will receive psychological support through every step of the journey [4].

With all this going on, how have you been coping?

- May I ask if you take alcohol in excess?
- May I ask if you take any recreational drugs?

Psychiatric History
Have you seen a psychiatrist in the past?

Family History
Anyone in the family with any mental or physical health issues?

Medication and Compliance
Do you take any regular medication?
    Do you take the medication as prescribed?

Brief Mental State Examination

Ask about mood, sleep, appetite, anhedonia, generalised anxiety, and auditory and visual hallucinations.

Risk Assessment

Suicidal thoughts or plans, thoughts of harming others and deliberate self-harm [1].

Station-Specific Points

Clarify how the individual would like to be addressed at the start of the assessment.

Generalised Anxiety Disorder

Scenario

31-year-old David Smith has been feeling increasingly anxious and has been referred by the GP to psychiatric services.

Task

Take a history.

Approach

Hello, I am Dr. ____. I am a psychiatrist. I understand you have been having some difficulties. I am sorry to hear that. Please could you tell me more?

History of Presenting Complaint
- May I ask what difficulties you are experiencing?
- When did this all first start?
- What was happening in your life at that time?
- How has this progressed?
- What kind of things make you anxious?
- When you do feel anxious, how long does this feeling last?
- How often in the course of a day can you feel this way?
- How do you feel between episodes?
- Anything that makes these feelings better or worse?
- Are there any stressors in your life?
- How would you describe your personality [1]?

Elicit the Symptoms Associated with Generalised Anxiety Disorder
- When you feel anxious, what kind of things do you experience in your body—heart racing, shortness of breath, sweating and dry mouth?
- And when you feel this way, what thoughts run through your mind: Do you worry something awful will happen, or do you worry about losing control [5]?

Impact and Coping

This sounds really difficult for you. How has this impacted on your

- Relationships
- Work

With all this going on, how have you been coping?

- May I ask if you take alcohol in excess?
- May I ask if you take any recreational drugs?

Psychiatric History

Have you seen a psychiatrist in the past?

Family History

Anyone in the family with any mental or physical health issues?

Medication and Compliance

Do you take any regular medication?
   Do you take the medication as prescribed?

Brief Mental State Examination

Ask about mood, sleep, appetite, anhedonia, and auditory and visual hallucinations.

Risk Assessment

Suicidal thoughts or plans, thoughts of harming others and deliberate self-harm

Differential Diagnosis

- Do you worry when you have to go to crowded places?
- Do you get anxious when you have to give a presentation?
- Do you have any specific fears—heights or closed spaces?
- Do you have any excessive checking or washing behaviours [1]?

Social Anxiety Disorder

Scenario

27-year-old Francesca Bolton was referred by the GP. She is due to get married and has been feeling increasingly anxious.

Task

Take a history.

Approach

Hello, I am Dr. _____. I am a psychiatrist. I understand you have been having some difficulties. I am sorry to hear that. Please could you tell me more?

History of Presenting Complaint
- May I ask what difficulties you are experiencing?
- When did this all first start?
- What was happening in your life at that time?
- How has this progressed?
- What kind of things make you anxious?
- When you do feel anxious, how long does this feeling last?
- How often in the course of a day can you feel this way?
- How do you feel between episodes?
- Anything that makes these feelings better or worse?
- Are there any stressors in your life?
- How would you describe your personality [1]?

Elicit the Physical and Psychological Symptoms
- When you feel anxious, what kind of things do you experience in your body— heart racing, shortness of breath, sweating and dry mouth?
- And when you feel this way, what thoughts run through your mind: Do you worry something awful will happen, or do you worry about losing control?
- Do you feel anxious in social situations?
- Avoidance: Do you try to avoid situations that make you anxious?
- Anticipatory anxiety: Do you worry in anticipation of an upcoming social event like your wedding [6]?

Impact and Coping

This sounds really difficult for you. How has this impacted on your

- Relationships
- Work
- Do you think you have chosen a line of work that limits social interactions?
- Do you think you are working below your capabilities due to being anxious?

   With all this going on, how have you been coping?

- May I ask if you take alcohol in excess?
- May I ask if you take any recreational drugs?

Psychiatric History

Have you seen a psychiatrist in the past?

Family History

Anyone in the family with any mental or physical health issues?

Medication and Compliance

Do you take any regular medication?
   Do you take the medication as prescribed?

Brief Mental State Examination

Ask about mood, sleep, appetite, anhedonia, and auditory and visual hallucinations.

Risk Assessment

Suicidal thoughts or plans, thoughts of harming others and deliberate self-harm

Differential Diagnosis

- Do you worry about everyday things?
- Do you worry when you have to go to crowded places?
- Do you have any specific fears—heights or closed spaces?
- Do you have any excessive checking or washing behaviours [1]?

Station-Specific Points

- Enquire about avoidance and anticipatory anxiety.

Panic Disorder

Scenario

26-year-old William Shelley has been having discrete periods of extreme anxiety and has been referred by the GP.

Task

Take a history and explain the diagnosis.

Approach

Hello, I am Dr. _____. I am a psychiatrist. I understand you have been having some difficulties. I am sorry to hear that. Please could you tell me more?

History of Presenting Complaint
- May I ask what difficulties you are experiencing?
- When did this all first start?
- What was happening in your life at that time?
- How has this progressed?
- What kind of things make you anxious?
- When you do feel anxious, how long does this feeling last?
- How often in the course of a day can you feel this way?
- How do you feel between episodes?
- Anything that makes these feelings better or worse?
- Are there any stressors in your life?
- How would you describe your personality [1]?

Elicit the Physical and Psychological Symptoms
- When you feel anxious, what kind of things do you experience in your body—heart racing, shortness of breath, sweating and dry mouth?
- And when you feel this way, what thoughts run through mind: Do you worry something awful will happen, or do you worry about losing control?
- Avoidance: Do you try to avoid things that might make you anxious?
- Anticipatory anxiety: Do you worry about when the next episode may occur [7]?

Impact and Coping
This sounds really difficult for you. How has this impacted on your

- Relationships
- Work

With all this going on, how have you been coping?

- May I ask if you take alcohol in excess?
- May I ask if you take any recreational drugs at all?
- May I ask if you take caffeine in any form—coffee or energy drinks?

Psychiatric History

Have you seen a psychiatrist in the past?

Family History

Anyone in the family with any mental or physical health issues?

Medication and Compliance

Do you take any regular medication?
    Do you take the medication as prescribed?

Brief Mental State Examination

Ask about mood, sleep, appetite, anhedonia, and auditory and visual hallucinations.

Risk Assessment

Suicidal thoughts or plans, thoughts of harming others and deliberate self-harm

Differential Diagnosis

- Do you worry about everyday things?
- Do you get anxious when you have to give a presentation?
- Do you worry when you have to go to crowded places?
- Do you have any specific fears—heights or closed spaces?
- Do you have any excessive checking or washing behaviours [1]?

Explain the Diagnosis

From our discussion today, it appears that the most likely diagnosis is panic disorder. This is a condition where the person experiences unexpected discrete periods of intense anxiety and panic. In most cases, there is no obvious trigger for feeling this way. It is accompanied by a persistent worry of the next episode and avoidance of situations that might precipitate this [7].

Station-Specific Points

Enquire about onset, duration and progression.

Epilepsy

Scenario

24-year-old Shaun Williams has been diagnosed with depression and started on tra-zodone by the GP. Recently, the dose was increased following which he had episodes where he stares into space for a few minutes without being aware he is doing this.

Task

Take a collateral history from his mother Mrs. Williams and identify possible aetiological factors.

Approach

Hello, I am Dr. _____. I am a psychiatrist. I understand your son Shaun has been having some difficulties. I am sorry to hear that. Please could you tell me more?

History of Presenting Complaint
- When did you first notice this?
- What was happening in his life at that time?
- Has anything like this happened before?
- Did this start suddenly or gradually?
- How has this progressed?
- Anything that makes it better or worse [1]?

Elicit the Symptoms of Epilepsy
- How often do the episodes occur?
- How long do the episodes last?
- Do they start in one part of the body and spread to the rest of the body?
- During the episode, does he experience any limb jerking, tongue biting, and incontinence of urine or faeces?
- Is he able to remember what happens during the episode?
- Does he feel his hair standing on end during the episode?

Aura
During the episode, does he have any unusual experiences like
- Hearing a buzzing noise
- Distortion of shape and size of various objects
- Odd sensations in his tummy

Altered Consciousness
- Does he have a motionless stare during the episode?
- Does he remain unresponsive to questions during the episode?

Automatisms
- Does he demonstrate any lip smacking, chewing, swallowing movements or hand movements [8]?

Impact and Coping
This sounds really difficult for Shaun. How has this impacted on his

- Relationships
- Work
- Driving

With all this going on, how has he been coping?

- May I ask if he takes alcohol in excess?
- May I ask if he takes any recreational drugs?

Psychiatric History
Have you seen a psychiatrist in the past?

Family History
Anyone in the family with seizures or febrile seizures?

Medical History
Any recent infections or head injury?

Medication and Compliance
Does he take any regular medication?
   Have there been any recent changes in the dose?

Brief Mental State Examination
Ask about mood, sleep, appetite, anhedonia, generalised anxiety, and auditory and visual hallucinations.

Risk Assessment
- Suicidal thoughts or plans, thoughts of harming others and deliberate self-harm
- Driving [1]

Station-Specific Points

- Identify whether the increase in medication trazodone has led to the current presentation [9].
- Remember to ask about driving risk.
- Discuss voluntarily informing driver and vehicle licensing agency.

Metabolic Syndrome

Scenario

44-year-old George Smith has been on clozapine for the last 6 years. His most recent clozapine monitoring bloods show increased triglyceride levels, low HDL cholesterol levels, increased fasting glucose levels, elevated blood pressure and increased waist circumference.

Task

Discuss the test results, explain the diagnosis and devise a management plan.

Approach

Hello, I am Dr. _____. I am a psychiatrist. I understand you are on clozapine, and we are here to discuss the results of the recent tests you had.

Before I explain the results, I would like to ask you a few questions please:

- Have there ever been any issues with any previous test results?
- Have you noticed an increase in your weight recently?
- Do you feel more thirsty?
- Do you feel like you have to wee more often?
- Family history of heart disease, hypertension and diabetes?
- Do you smoke?
- Do you take alcohol?
- Do you have a sedentary lifestyle?
- How have you found being on clozapine?

Explain Metabolic Syndrome
- The test results show that you have increased blood sugar levels, decreased HDL cholesterol or healthy fat levels, increased triglycerides or unhealthy fat levels, along with an elevated blood pressure and increase in your waist circumference.
- This combination is called metabolic syndrome.

- Have you heard of this before?
- This is a side effect of being on antipsychotic medication like clozapine.
- The frequency of metabolic syndrome is five times higher in individuals with schizophrenia.

Management
1. We will refer to the GP.
2. Further testing of increased blood sugar levels and prescribing medication to reduce blood sugar levels if necessary.
3. Monitoring of blood pressure. Prescribing medication to reduce blood pressure if necessary.
4. Medication called statins can be prescribed to control increased levels of unhealthy fats.
5. Regular checks of blood pressure and blood tests.
6. Referral to dietician.
7. Diet modification: diet low in saturated fats with plenty of fruits and vegetables.
8. Regular exercise for at least 30 min a day, five times a week.
9. Smoking cessation and limiting alcohol consumption.
10. Switching medication is not recommended at present and will only be considered after all the above methods have been tried and have been unsuccessful.
11. Increased blood sugar levels can lead to complications; therefore, it is important to manage elevated levels appropriately.

Station-Specific Points

- Explain the adverse effects of high blood sugars.
- Explain that clozapine will be changed only as a last resort [10].

Serotonin Syndrome

Scenario

22-year-old Jack Shelby has been on fluoxetine and showed a partial response; therefore, his medication was changed to sertraline following which he began feeling unwell with tachycardia, hyperthermia, vomiting, confusion and agitation. He is currently admitted in hospital. His mother Mrs. Shelby is waiting to speak to you.

Task

Explain the diagnosis and devise a management plan.

Approach

Hello, I am Dr. _____. I am a psychiatrist. I understand you are waiting to speak to me about Jack. Please may I clarify what your understanding is of what is happening with Jack. It appears that he has developed a condition called serotonin syndrome. Have you heard of this before?

Explain Serotonin Syndrome
- Serotonin syndrome is a condition that occurs when there is too much of a chemical called serotonin in the brain.
- Serotonin is the chemical that controls mood, temperature and how fast your heart beats among other things. The medication used to treat depression increases the levels of serotonin in the brain; however, following the recent change in medication, it appears that he has developed serotonin syndrome as a result of too much serotonin.

Management
1. The antidepressant medication that has caused this condition has been stopped.
2. He has to remain in the medical hospital where the staff are trained to manage medical conditions.
3. There will be continuous monitoring of his blood pressure, heart rate, breathing and other vital signs.
4. He will receive supportive treatment like intravenous fluids.
5. Once he is completely well, we will slowly restart on antidepressant medication while closely monitoring for any adverse reactions.
6. We will make a clear entry in his notes of his current presentation.
7. Prognosis: He has been diagnosed quickly and is receiving appropriate care and treatment. Therefore, the prognosis is good. It is unlikely that there will be any permanent damage [11].

Antidepressant-Induced Side Effects

Scenario

45-year-old Thomas MacPherson was started on citalopram a few weeks ago and has been referred by the GP since he has been having some side effects and wants to stop medication.

Task

Devise a management plan.

Approach

Hello, I am Dr. _____. I am a psychiatrist. I understand you have been having some side effects.

I understand you have been prescribed citalopram:

- What dose are you on?
- How long have you been taking this medication?
- Have you been taking the medication regularly?
- Have you experienced any side effects?
- If you do not mind me asking, some people experience issues during intimacy while on this medication—have you had any issues?
- Sexual difficulties can be a side effect of medication and we can address this.

I need to ask you a few personal questions:

- How has your interest in sex been?
- Are you able to get an erection?
- Are you able to maintain an erection?
- Do you ejaculate too quickly?
- Do you have an early-morning erection?
- Did you have any of these difficulties prior to starting citalopram?

Physical Causes

- Do you have diabetes, underactive thyroid and recent surgeries?
- Are you on any other medication?

Alcohol and Substance Misuse

- Do you use alcohol in excess?
- Do you take any recreational drugs?

Psychiatric Causes

- Depressive symptoms: Ask about mood, sleep appetite, anhedonia, energy levels and concentration.
- Do you have any unusual experiences like hearing voices or seeing things when there is no one else around?
- Do you tend to be generally anxious?
- Thoughts of harming yourself or others?

Social Causes

- Do you have any marital issues?
- How is your intimate relationship?
- Do you experience performance anxiety?
- Environment at home—lack of privacy or worry that someone may walk in during intimate moments?
- Do you have any stress in your life or work?

Management

1. Stopping medication is not advisable as there is a risk that the depressive symptoms may worsen and you could relapse.
2. Watchful waiting: In 5–10% of cases, the side effects can subside spontaneously in a few months.
3. We can consider reducing the current dose and monitor carefully.
4. Drug holidays of one or two days prior to sexual intercourse.
5. Discontinue this medication and switch to a different medication like mirtazapine.
6. Medication like Viagra can be used as required to treat antidepressant-induced erectile dysfunction.
7. Talking therapy to address any marital issues.
8. I will request GP to do some blood tests including thyroid function tests and checking the levels of a chemical called prolactin.
9. With your permission, I can speak to your partner [12].

Station-Specific Points

Explore sexual history in a sensitive manner.

Abnormal Grief Reaction

Scenario

67-year-old Beatrice Wilson has recently lost her husband. She has been referred to your clinic by the GP as he is concerned with her presentation.

Task

Assess her to distinguish between normal and abnormal grief reaction.

Approach

Hello, I am Dr. _____. I am a psychiatrist. I understand you have lost your spouse recently. I am sorry to hear about your loss.

- When did you lose your spouse?
- Please can you tell me about the circumstances leading to your spouse's demise?
- Were you with your spouse at that time?
- Did you have any form of closure?
- Did you attend the wake?
- Have you been to visit the grave since then?
- How was your relationship with your spouse?
- Do you feel angry?
- Do you blame anyone for your spouse's demise?
- Have you had times when you were bargaining, wishing it were you instead of your spouse?
- Have you left your spouse's belongings as though he/she were still in the house?
- Do you feel you are slowly coming to terms with your loss?
- Do you feel you are at a place where you accept that he/she is no more [13]?

Impact and Coping

This sounds really difficult for you. How has this impacted on your

- Relationships
- Work
- Finances
- Ability to care for family

With all this going on, how have you been coping?

- May I ask if you take alcohol in excess?
- May I ask if you take any recreational drugs?

Brief Mental State Examination

- Explore mood, sleep, appetite, energy, anhedonia and self-neglect.
- Are there times you feel you can still hear or see your spouse?
- Do you hear any other voices?
- Do you see anything else?
- Do you feel responsible for your spouse's death?
- Do have any thoughts of ending your life?

Psychiatric History

Have you seen a psychiatrist in the past?

Family History

Anyone in the family with any mental or physical health issues [1]?

Station-Specific Points

- Elicit information about stages of grief, denial, anger, bargaining, depression and acceptance.
- Be sensitive and empathic in your approach.

Mania Management

Scenario

23-year-old Ryan Russell has been brought to the GP by his concerned parents. He has been elated with increased energy and has not slept in 3 days. He had a similar presentation 2 years ago and was treated with lithium; however, he recently stopped his medication. The GP has given Ryan some medication to calm him and referred for urgent psychiatric review.

Task

Explain the diagnosis and devise a management plan.

Approach

Hello, I am Dr. _____. I am a psychiatrist. I understand you have been having some difficulties.

- From the information available, I understand that you have increased energy with little sleep and you are extremely happy. You have some grand plans. All these symptoms suggest that you are experiencing a manic episode similar to what you have previously experienced 2 years ago. It indicates a diagnosis of bipolar affective disorder. May I ask if you have heard of this before?
- We all experience minor changes in our mood from one day to the next as an appropriate response to life events. However, people with bipolar affective disorder have major mood swings alternating between being very happy and sad for no obvious reason.
- Fortunately, we can reduce or even prevent further episodes with regular medication.

I am aware you were on lithium previously:

- May I ask why you stopped taking it?
- Any side effects?

Management

1. We will urgently check your lithium level, and if you are willing, we can restart lithium.
2. We can start antipsychotic medication like olanzapine.
3. I will check with your parents; however, if you take your medication regularly, have support at home and do not present a significant risk to yourself or others, it would be reasonable for you to continue as an outpatient.
4. A community psychiatric nurse will pay you weekly visits to offer intensive support.
5. Please take time off work if you do work.
6. If your condition worsens and your parents or the nurse expresses concerns, we will have to consider hospital admission [14].

Neuroleptic Malignant Syndrome

Scenario

20-year-old Harris Wiles was admitted to the psychiatric hospital 2 days ago with psychotic symptoms. He was very aggressive on the ward and received haloperidol 5 mg on two separate occasions. Soon after the second injection, he developed hyperthermia, severe muscle rigidity, confusion, tachycardia and hypertension. Blood tests show elevated creatine phosphokinase. You are speaking to his father Mr. Wiles.

Task

Explain the diagnosis.
   Discuss the management plan.

Approach

Hello, I am Dr. ____. I am a psychiatrist. I understand we are here to discuss your son Harris.

Explain Neuroleptic Malignant Syndrome

- I am sorry to say that your son appears to have developed a rare condition called neuroleptic malignant syndrome, which is an unpredictable side effect of antipsychotic medication that was given to him.
- It presents with high temperature, muscle stiffness, confusion with changes in blood pressure and changes in pulse rate.
- This medication was used according to hospital policy to manage the situation to ensure the safety of your son and the people around him.

Management

1. This is a medical emergency.
2. Firstly, we have stopped the antipsychotic immediately.
3. Transferred to the medical intensive care unit as it is the best place for him.
4. Continuous monitoring of vital signs—temperature, blood pressure and pulse.
5. Blood tests including full blood count, kidney function test, liver function test and levels of a chemical called creatine kinase that is elevated in this condition.
6. Further investigations like electrical tracing of the heart.
7. Rehydration with fluids and medication to help control symptoms including correction of salt imbalances.
8. After about 2 weeks, once he is fully recovered, we will consider restarting the antipsychotic medication.
9. We will begin with a small dose and increase slowly.
10. We will avoid depots and typical type of antipsychotics like haloperidol.
11. We will involve you and your son in the decision-making process.
12. We will clearly document in the notes regarding adverse reaction to the medication used.
13. We will use a multidisciplinary team approach involving the medical team and psychiatrists.
    - This condition can be life-threatening with a 10% risk; however, we have recognised the condition early; he is in the right place and will receive all the appropriate treatment therefore the outcome is good.
    - Differential diagnosis—malignant hyperthermia and meningitis.
    - Complications—kidney or heart complications.
    - If you wish to complain, I can refer you to the patient advisory liaison service [15].

Station-Specific Points

- Clearly mention it is a medical emergency.
- First step is to stop the antipsychotic medication.
- Anticipate that the actor may be angry.

Hyperprolactinemia

Scenario

30-year-old Jane Patters has been on risperidone 6 mg for schizophrenia with mental health stable on medication. Blood test done at the GP practice shows a prolactin level of 100 ng/mL (normal range in women 0–25 ng/mL).

Task

Explain the results.
   Discuss the management plan.

Approach

Hello, I am Dr. _____. I am a psychiatrist. I understand you are here to discuss the blood test results.

- Unfortunately, the results are abnormal and show an increase in the levels of a chemical called prolactin.
- This is a side effect of risperidone.

  May I ask you a few personal questions please?
  Have you noticed any

- Breast enlargement
- Discharge from your breast
- Changes in your desire for sex
- Changes in your menstrual cycle
- Lumps in your breast
- Headaches or blurring of vision

  All of these symptoms are related to the raised levels of prolactin.
  In the long term, it might cause

- Thinning of the bones
- Increase in the risk of developing breast cancer

Management
1. Switch to another antipsychotic that does not increase prolactin levels like olanzapine or quetiapine.
2. Add another antipsychotic, namely aripiprazole, to reduce the levels of prolactin.

3. Increase weight-bearing exercise, adequate calcium and vitamin D3 intake.
4. Psychoeducation.
5. Information leaflets [16].

Bipolar Affective Disorder: Depression—Discussion and Management

Scenario

29-year-old Alexander Bain was admitted to hospital under the mental health act after experiencing a manic episode and started on risperidone. After 4 weeks of treatment, the manic symptoms improved; however, he started displaying symptoms consistent with depression for which he was started on citalopram with poor response.

Task

Explain the most likely diagnosis and discuss management with her.

Approach

Hello, I am Dr. _____. I am a psychiatrist. I understand you were admitted to hospital 4 weeks ago with a manic episode started on medication and improved and however subsequently developed symptoms suggestive of depression for which we started on medication with limited improvement.

- May I check how your mood is now?
- How are your energy levels?
- How is your sleep?
- How is your appetite?
- Do you still feel able to enjoy the activities you previously enjoyed?
- How is your memory?
- How is your concentration?
- How is your motivation?
- How is your self-esteem?
- How do you see the future?
- Do you have any suicidal thoughts or suicidal plans?
- Do you have any thoughts of harming yourself [17]?

Based on the information we have so far, it would appear that you are having a condition called bipolar affective disorder.

We all experience minor changes in our mode from one day to the next as an appropriate response to life events. People with bipolar affective disorder have major mood changes alternating between being very happy and very depressed for no obvious reason.

In your case, you started with a manic episode and then subsequently became depressed, which is indicative of bipolar affective disorder with a depressive episode at present.

Management

1. Fluoxetine is the antidepressant recommended according to the National Institute for Health and Care Excellence guidelines to treat the depressive symptoms.
2. In addition, an antipsychotic like olanzapine can be used.
3. Alternatively, lamotrigine may be considered. This needs to be started on a low dose and slowly increased. It can also have side effect of a skin rash called Stevens-Johnson syndrome.
4. Another option is lithium, which is a mood stabiliser. This involves regular weekly blood testing to ensure that lithium is within the treatment range and other tests as well [18].

What are your thoughts about the medication options we have discussed?

I will see you again to discuss further if you have any queries or require further information.

Depression and Myocardial Infarction

Scenario

59-year-old Anne Wagner had a recent myocardial infarction and is currently admitted in the cardiology ward. She has a previous diagnosis of depression treated with cognitive behavioural therapy. At present time, she describes low mood, poor sleep and appetite with poor motivation. She denies any thoughts of wanting to harm herself; however, she feels hopeless about the future. At the request of the cardiology consultant, you have spoken to the patient already.

Task

Speak to the medical student Jason Parker on the cardiology ward and answer his questions about this patient.

Approach

I am Dr. ___. I am a psychiatrist. I have reviewed Mrs. Wagner and understand you have a few questions for me.

Q1. What do you think is the diagnosis?

A1. Based on the fact that she is describing low mood, poor sleep and appetite, and poor motivation and however denies any thoughts of wanting to harm herself with feelings of hopelessness about the future, the most likely diagnosis is mild-to-moderate depression.

Q2. What medication would you be considering?

A2. I would be considering sertraline.

Q3. Are there any medication you would avoid?

A3. I would avoid tricyclic antidepressants and monoamine oxidase inhibitors, which can precipitate arrhythmias. I would use fluoxetine with caution due to enzyme-inhibiting effect on cytchrome P450 system and potential to interact with cardiac medication. I would also exercise caution if using venlafaxine due to the effect on blood pressure.

Q4. Do you think the myocardial infarction has caused the depression or the depression has caused the myocardial infarction?

A4. This is a difficult question to answer. Physical health issues can cause a person to become depressed. Conversely, being depressed makes it less likely that the person would have the motivation to engage in exercise, follow a healthy diet and engage with any treatment plan, which makes them more susceptible to develop physical health problems.

Q5. Do you think cognitive behavioural therapy would be useful now?

A5. Given the current presentation, I would start with medication, and cognitive behavioural therapy can be considered at a later stage.

Q6. What are your long-term recommendations?

A6. I would suggest a multidisciplinary team approach with regular psychiatric review, psychoeducation and support to patient and family [19].

Q7. Would you consider electroconvulsive therapy?

A7. Electroconvulsive therapy is relatively contraindicated in patients who have had a myocardial infarction in the last 3 months. However, if the patient is not responding to medication or if there are concerns for his safety, it can be considered as a last resort after anaesthetist opinion. It is administered in a special hospital suite, which has cardiac resuscitation facilities [20].

Station-Specific Points

- Answer the questions posed by the role player to progress through the station.
- Medical jargon can be used as you are speaking to a medical colleague.

Depression

Scenario

44-year-old Paul Bernard has a diagnosis of depression and is on treatment with venlafaxine 225 mg for 2 months with a partial response. He has previously been tried on fluoxetine with limited benefit.

Task

Take a brief history to identify reasons for the lack of response and formulate a management plan.

Approach

I am Dr. ___. I am a psychiatrist. I understand you are having a few difficulties.

Symptoms of Depression
Ask about mood, sleep, appetite, anhedonia, energy levels, memory, concentration, motivation and suicidal thoughts.

Medical History
Enquire about symptoms of hypothyroidism—constipation, weight gain, sensitivity to cold weather and hair loss.
    Enquire about heart problems, high blood pressure, epilepsy and diabetes.

Psychiatric History
Ask about generalised anxiety, hearing voices, seeing things and feeling elated.

Medication
Current medication, recent changes in any medication and compliance

Alcohol/Substance Misuse
- Do you take alcohol in excess?
- Do you take recreational drugs?

Stressors
Anything in your life causing you stress [1]?

Management
1. Optimise the dose of venlafaxine and increase to 300 mg.
2. Refer to the GP to regularly monitor blood pressure and pulse rate and take a tracing of your heart.

3. We can also consider talking therapy like cognitive behavioural therapy.
4. The standard treatment for depression according to the National Institute for Health and Care Excellence guidelines is to trial an antidepressant for 4–6 weeks. If there is insufficient response, we start an antidepressant from a different class and it is trialled over 4–6 weeks. If there is still no response, we consider a diagnosis of treatment-resistant depression.
5. The next step is augmenting antidepressant by adding lithium and in severe cases electroconvulsive therapy [21].

Station-Specific Points

Clarify that the diagnosis at present is not one of treatment-resistant depression as there is still scope to increase venlafaxine.

Treatment-Resistant Schizophrenia

Scenario

32-year-old Cody Jacobson has been an inpatient in a psychiatric ward for the last 3 months. He has been tried on two different antipsychotic medications with little effect. He was started on clozapine 1 week ago and appears to be a slow responder. His mother has come to visit him and would like to speak to you.

Task

Speak to Mrs. Jacobson and answer her queries.

Approach

I am Dr. _____ and I am a psychiatrist. I understand you visited your son today and you have a few questions for me.

Explain the Rationale for Starting Clozapine
- When two different antipsychotic medications have been tried with inadequate response, clozapine is initiated.
- Discuss the regular blood tests and monitoring of clozapine.
- Explain that there may be a delay in the onset of action—every individual is different and their responses also vary; some may respond sooner than others [22].
- Staying in hospital involves a lot more than just medication. There will be a range of professionals active in his care. He will have continuous supervision and will be carefully monitored.

- Inform about the hospital complaint procedure.
- Inform that the family can attend ward meetings for him and this will allow them to be involved in decisions made regarding his care.

Station-Specific Points

- Anticipate that the mother will be angry.
- Remain calm and confident.
- Be empathic and acknowledge her concerns.

Schizophrenia and Substance Misuse

Scenario

39-year-old Robert Clarke has a diagnosis of schizophrenia and is on risperidone 6 mg. The community psychiatric nurse has expressed concerns as he appears to have relapsed and is having mental health issues again.

Task

Take a brief history and discuss the management options.

Approach

Hello I am Dr. ____. I understand that the community psychiatric nurse has expressed concerns about your mental health.

Brief History and Mental State Examination
- How has your mood been?
- Have you seen things when there is no one around you?
- Have you heard voices when there is no one around you?
- Any thoughts of harming yourself or others?
- Do you have any medical problems?
- Are you taking your medication as prescribed?
- If compliance is poor: When did you stop taking the medication, why did you stop taking the medication and did you experience any side effects?
- Do you take any recreational drugs—clarify what he takes, how much and how often.
- Enquire about social support [1].

Management

1. Restart antipsychotic medication: We might consider aripiprazole that has less propensity for side effects. However, like any medication, it may have some side effects like feeling more sleepy and gaining weight.
2. I will refer to the substance misuse service to assist you with stopping cannabis use.
3. Inform if he can be managed in the community with input from the crisis team or whether he needs admission to the hospital. This decision will be based on social support, current mental health, risk assessment and willingness to engage with treatment plan [23].
4. I would advise that you stop using cannabis immediately—as it increases symptoms, impairs recovery and can interfere with the antipsychotic medication [24].

Station-Specific Points

Explain the effects of cannabis use on mental health.

Weight Gain Psychosocial History

Scenario

30-year-old Claire Forbes has a diagnosis of depression treated with venlafaxine. Due to partial response, the GP recently added mirtazapine. She has gained weight over the last year and is concerned about this.

Task

Take a psychosocial history.
Assess motivation to lose weight.

Approach

Hello I am Dr. ____. I understand you have started on mirtazapine and have concerns about weight gain.

- When were you started on mirtazapine?
- When did you start gaining weight?
- What was happening in your life at that time?
- How much exercise do you manage to get in a week?
- Do you think you have a healthy diet?
- Do you have a sedentary job?

- Do you drink alcohol—how much and how often?
- Do you take any recreational drugs?
- Do you have any medical problems—high blood pressure, diabetes and high cholesterol?
- Family history.
- The medication mirtazapine can cause weight gain as a side effect.

Explore the impact of weight gain on:

- Work
- Relationships
- Social life

Brief mental state examination:

- Mood
- Sleep
- Appetite
- Anhedonia
- Hearing voices/seeing things
- Thoughts of harming himself or others
- An increase in weight has a variety of implications on the overall health. It increases the chances of having heart problems like a heart attack or stroke [25].
- Do you think you need help to address your weight gain?
- Would you be willing to lose weight, stop smoking, decrease alcohol consumption or abstain, eat a healthy diet and exercise?
- How motivated are you to engage with this?

Station-Specific Points

Explore his motivation to engage in diet and exercise program for weight loss.

References

1. Semple D, Smyth R. Chapter 2. Psychiatric assessment. History. Mental state examination. Oxford handbook of psychiatry. 3rd ed. Oxford University Press; 2017. p. 42–44.
2. National Institute for Health and Care Excellence. Post- traumatic stress disorder NICE guideline [NG116]. 2018. https://www.nice.org.uk/guidance/ng116/chapter/Recommendations#recognition-of-post-traumatic-stress-disorder. Accessed 5 December.
3. World Health Organization. Obsessive-compulsive or related disorders (BlockL1-6B2). 6B20 Obsessive-compulsive disorder. ICD-11 International Classification of Diseases—mortality and morbidity statistics. 11th revision ed. World Health Organization; 2018. p. 43.
4. Royal College of Psychiatrists London. Good practice guidelines for the assessment and treatment of adults with gender dysphoria. College Report. 2013;CR181.

5. Semple D, Smyth R. Generalized anxiety disorder. Oxford handbook of psychiatry. 3rd ed. Oxford University Press; 2017. p. 372.

6. National Institute for Health and Care Excellence. Social anxiety disorder: recognition, assessment and treatment clinical guideline [CG159]. 2013. https://www.nice.org.uk/guidance/cg159/chapter/Recommendations#identification-and-assessment-of-adults-2. Accessed 22 May.

7. World Health Organization. Anxiety or fear-related disorders (BlockL1-6B0). 6B01 Panic disorder. ICD-11 International Classification of Diseases—mortality and morbidity statistics. 11th revision ed. World Health Organization; 2018. p. 40.

8. McIntosh W, Das J. Temporal seizure. 2022. https://www.ncbi.nlm.nih.gov/books/NBK549852/. Accessed July.

9. Hill T, Coupland C, Morriss R, Arthur A, Moore M, Hippisley-Cox J. Antidepressant use and risk of epilepsy and seizures in people aged 20 to 64 years: cohort study using a primary care database. BMC Psychiatry. 2015;15:315.

10. Ho C, Zhang M, Mak A, Ho R. Metabolic syndrome in psychiatry: advances in understanding and management. Adv Psychiatr Treat. 2014;20.

11. Wang R, Vashistha V, Kaur S, Houchens N. Serotonin syndrome: preventing, recognizing, and treating it. Cleve Clin J Med. 2016;83(11):810–7.

12. Taylor DM, Barnes T, Young A. Depression and anxiety disorders. Antidepressants and sexual dysfunction. The Maudsley prescribing guidelines in psychiatry. 14th ed. Wiley Blackwell; 2021. p. 404.

13. World Health Organization. Disorders specifically associated with stress (BlockL1-6B4). 6B42 Prolonged grief disorder. International Classification of Diseases—mortality and morbidity statistics. 11th revision ed. World Health Organization; 2019. p. 49.

14. National Institute for Health and Care Excellence. Bipolar disorder: assessment and management clinical guideline [CG185]. 2020. https://www.nice.org.uk/guidance/cg185/chapter/1-Recommendations#managing-bipolar-disorder-in-adults-in-the-longer-term-in-secondary-care-2. Accessed February.

15. Simon LV, Hashmi MF, Callahan AL. Neuroleptic malignant syndrome. 2022. https://www.ncbi.nlm.nih.gov/books/NBK482282/. Accessed August.

16. Taylor DM, Barnes T, Young A. Schizophrenia and related psychoses-antipsychotic adverse effects. The Maudsley prescribing guidelines in psychiatry. 14th ed. Wiley Blackwell; 2021. p. 168.

17. Casey P, Kelly B. Fish's clinical psychopathology signs and symptoms in psychiatry. 3rd ed. The Royal College of Psychiatrists; 2016.

18. Taylor DM, Barnes T, Young A. Bipolar disorder. Bipolar depression. The Maudsley prescribing guidelines in psychiatry. 14th ed. Wiley Blackwell; 2021. p. 288.

19. Taylor DM, Barnes T, Young A. Depression and anxiety disorders. Cardiac effects of antidepressants-summary. The Maudsley prescribing guidelines in psychiatry. 14th ed. Wiley Blackwell; 2021. p. 383.

20. Kho K. Depression post-myocardial infarction. Br J Psychiatry. 2007;191(5):456.

21. National Institute for Health and Care Excellence. Depression in adults: recognition and management. NICE guideline [NG222]. 2022. https://www.nice.org.uk/guidance/ng222/chapter/Recommendations#choice-of-treatments. Accessed June, NICE guideline [NG222].

22. Electronic Medicines Compendium (emc). Clozaril 100 mg tablets. https://www.medicines.org.uk/emc/product/10290/smpc.

23. Taylor DM, Barnes T, Young A. Schizophrenia and related psychoses. Antipsychotic drugs. The Maudsley prescribing guidelines in psychiatry. 14th ed. Wiley Blackwell; 2021. p. 3.

24. Semple D, Smyth R. Cannabis. Oxford handbook of psychiatry. 3rd ed. Oxford University Press; 2017. p. 588.

25. Sarwer D, Polonsky H. The psychosocial burden of obesity. Endocrinol Metab Clin North Am. 2016;45(3):677.

Dementia

Scenario

81-year-old Craig Hamilton has been referred by the GP since he has noticed a decline in his memory. There are concerns that he may be developing Alzheimer's dementia.

Task

Take a collateral history from his wife Patricia Hamilton and perform a risk assessment.

Approach

Hello, I am Dr. _____. I am a psychiatrist. I understand your husband has been having some difficulties with his memory. Please could you tell me more?

History of Presenting Complaint
- When did you first start noticing problems?
- What was happening in his life at that time?
- Did it start gradually or suddenly?
- How has it progressed?

All names and scenarios mentioned in this book are fictitious. Any resemblance to actual individuals or backgrounds is entirely conincidental.

© The Author(s), under exclusive license to Springer Nature
Switzerland AG 2023
N. Sivaswamy, *Prepare for the MRCPsych CASC Exam*,
https://doi.org/10.1007/978-3-031-31019-5_2

- Was it a sudden decline or a stepwise decline?
- What problems have you noticed?
- Does he forget people's names?
- Does he forget appointments?
- Does he forget conversations?
- Does he remember events from a few years ago?
- Does he lose his way around the neighbourhood?
- Does he know the date and day of the week?
- Does he have difficulty recognising objects?
- Does he have difficulty recognising familiar faces?
- Does he have word finding difficulties?
- Does he have difficulty understanding when someone speaks to him?
- Does he have difficulty looking after himself like personal hygiene, shopping and laundry?
- Does he have difficulty cooking a meal?
- Does he have difficulty organising bill to be paid or handling finances?
- Does he have difficulty solving everyday problems he used to be able to solve?
- How are his planning and decision-making abilities?

Personality
- Has he been more irritable recently?
- Any change in personality?
- Any aggressive episodes?
- Has he been socially withdrawn?
- Any socially inappropriate behaviour?

Physical Health
Does he have any

- Hearing or vision impairments
- Weakness of arms or legs
- Changes in the way he walks
- Unusual movements of his body
- Incontinence
- Sleep disturbances
- Appetite disturbances
- Weight loss

Impact and Coping
This sounds really difficult for you. How has this impacted on you and how are you coping?

Substance and Alcohol Misuse
May I ask if he takes alcohol in excess?
    May I ask if he takes any recreational drugs?

Psychiatric History

Has he seen a psychiatrist in the past?

Medical History
- Stroke
- High blood pressure
- Diabetes
- Fits
- Infections
- Thyroid disorders
- Head injury
- Constipation

Family History
- Anyone in the family with any mental or physical health issues?
- Anyone in the family with dementia?

Medication and Compliance

Do you take any regular medication?

Brief Mental State Examination

Ask about mood, sleep, appetite, anhedonia, generalised anxiety, auditory and visual hallucinations and insight.

Risk Assessment
- Suicidal thoughts or plans, thoughts of harming others and deliberate self-harm
- Self-neglect
- Inappropriate use for medication
- Falls
- Wandering
- Fire risk
- Driving risk
- Mismanagement of finances
- Aggression
- Carers' strain [1]

Station-Specific Points

This is a long station, so make judicious use of time.

Wandering Behaviour

Scenario

78-year-old Jeanne Rankin was found by the police wandering the streets. You have been asked by A&E to review this lady.

Task

Take a collateral history from his daughter Melissa Coffey.

Approach

Hello, I am Dr. ____. I am a psychiatrist. I understand your mother has been admitted to the hospital as she was found wandering around by the police. Please may I ask you a few questions?

Explore Details of the Incident
- What happened?
- Where was she found wandering?
- How was she found?
- Was she dressed appropriately?
- Any similar issues previously?
- Does she usually visit the place where she was found wandering?
- Have you noticed any issues with Jeanne that have concerned you?
- Is there anything stressful going on in her life?
- Did it start gradually or suddenly?
- How has it progressed?
- Was it a sudden decline or a stepwise decline?
- Have you noticed any issues with her memory?
- Does she forget people's names?
- Does she forget appointments?
- Does she forget conversations?
- Does she remember events from a few years ago?
- Does she lose her way around the neighbourhood?
- Does she have difficulty looking after herself like personal hygiene, shopping and laundry?
- Does she have difficulty cooking a meal?
- Does she have difficulty organising bill to be paid or handling finances?

Personality
- Has she been more irritable recently?
- Any change in personality?

- Any aggressive episodes?
- Has she been socially withdrawn?

Physical Health

Does she have any

- Hearing or vision impairments
- Weakness of arms or legs
- Changes in the way she walks
- Unusual movements of her body
- Incontinence

Explore Reasons for Wandering

- Do you think she might have gone there as she was bored?
- Could it have been habit?
- Could it have been a need for exercise?

Impact and Coping

This sounds really difficult for you. How has this impacted on you and how are you coping?

Substance and Alcohol Misuse

- May I ask if she takes alcohol in excess?
- May I ask if she takes any recreational drugs?

Psychiatric History

- Has she seen a psychiatrist in the past?

Medical History

Does she have

- Stroke
- High blood pressure
- Diabetes
- Fits
- Infections
- Thyroid disorders
- Head injury
- Constipation

Family History

- Anyone in the family with any mental or physical health issues?
- Anyone in the family with dementia?

Medication and Compliance
Does she take any regular medication?

Brief MSE
Ask about mood, sleep, appetite, anhedonia, generalised anxiety, auditory and visual hallucinations and insight.

Risk Assessment
- Suicidal thoughts or plans, thoughts of harming others and deliberate self-harm
- Self-neglect
- Inappropriate use of medication
- Falls
- Fire risk
- Driving risk
- Mismanagement of finances
- Aggression [2]

Vascular Dementia Management

Scenario

73-year-old John has been diagnosed with vascular dementia after having extensive investigations including CT brain scan. You are about to speak to his daughter.

Task

Speak to his daughter Jennifer, explain the diagnosis and management and answer her queries.

Approach

Hello, I am Dr. _____. I am a psychiatrist. I understand your father recently had tests for memory problems. May I please check what information you have so far?

Explain Vascular Dementia
- He appears to have a condition called vascular dementia. Have you heard of this before?
- Vascular dementia is a common form of dementia that occurs in people over the age of 70 years.
- It occurs because the blood vessels in the brain are diseased and over the years there is less blood reaching the brain resulting in strokes.
- This will lead to a stepwise decline in the person's physical health and cause memory problems.

- It is a progressive disease.

Risk Factors

- Smoking which leads to disease of the blood vessels
- High blood pressure
- High levels of unhealthy fats or cholesterol in the blood
- Diabetes or high blood sugar
- Heart disease
- Family history of vascular dementia

Diagnosis

Diagnosis is based on detailed clinical history, physical examination and investigations including imaging like CT/MRI brain [3].

Management

1. Antidementia medication is not useful.
2. Risk factor modification.
3. Antihypertensive medication to reduce blood pressure.
4. Statins to lower cholesterol levels.
5. If appropriate, use of blood thinners like aspirin to reduce the risk of stroke.
6. Treatment of underlying conditions like heart disease.
7. Lifestyle modification—balanced diet with plenty of fruits and vegetables that is low in saturated fats.
8. Smoking cessation—we can offer help with this if required.
9. Limit or abstain from alcohol use.
10. Keeping the brain active by doing puzzles, sudoku and reading.
11. Carers' support and respite care.
12. Leaflets.
13. Support groups [1].

Lewy Body Dementia Management

Scenario

75-year-old Tony has been diagnosed with Lewy body dementia. You are about to speak to his son.

Task

Speak to his son, explain the diagnosis and further management and answer his queries.

Approach

Hello, I am Dr. ___. I am a psychiatrist. I understand your father recently had tests for memory problems. May I please check what information you have so far?

Explain Lewy Body Dementia
- He appears to have a condition called Lewy body dementia. Have you heard of this before?
- It is a type of dementia associated with the presence of protein deposits called Lewy bodies in the brain that disturb its normal functioning.

It presents with

- Movement problems like shakiness and muscle stiffness
- Seeing things that are not really there
- Changes in alertness levels
- Increased sensitivity to some medication
- It is a progressive disease with a steady decline in memory and brain function [4].

Medication will help slow the decline.

The Difference Between Lewy Body Dementia and Parkinson's Dementia
- In Lewy body dementia, the movement problems and memory issues both develop within 12 months.
- In Parkinson's, the movement issues have existed for over 12 months before the memory issues develop.

Dopamine Transporter Scan
It is a special scan used to differentiate between Lewy body dementia and Alzheimer's dementia. However, the scan cannot differentiate between Lewy body dementia and Parkinson's dementia.

The diagnosis remains a clinical one with investigations and blood tests that help exclude other causes.

Management
1. It is important to weigh up the risks and benefits and use a balanced approach while prescribing medication.
2. Antiparkinsonian medication can be used to treat the movement problems.
3. Antidementia medication like rivastigmine may be used (despite not being licensed for treating Lewy body dementia) and is useful in individuals with visual hallucinations and challenging behaviours.
4. Common side effects of this medication are feeling sick, vomiting and loose stools.

5. Antipsychotic medication is used with extreme caution as they can worsen movement problems as individuals with Lewy body dementia are sensitive to this medication.
6. Psychological therapy—psychoeducation, reassurance and support, reminiscence therapy and reality orientation.
7. Multidisciplinary team approach—community psychiatric nurse, occupational therapist, physiotherapist and neurologist.
8. Carers' assessment.
9. Ambulatory aids—Zimmer frames and walking stick.
10. Carers' support and respite care.
11. Leaflets.
12. Support groups [1].

Station-Specific Points

- Chunk and check
- Follow a biopsychosocial approach while explaining management

---

Mania: Medication Induced

Scenario

Charlie Hammersmith is 75 years old with a diagnosis of Parkinson's disease. He is on treatment with levodopa and resides at a care home. The staff have been expressing concerns about his behaviour for the last 1 week.

Task

Take a history, and identify possible etiological factors and the most likely diagnosis.

Approach

Hello, I am Dr. ____. I am a psychiatrist. I understand that care home staff have expressed some concerns about you.

History of Presenting Complaint
- May I ask what difficulties you are experiencing?
- When did this all first start?
- What was happening in your life at that time?
- How has this progressed?
- Anything that makes these feelings better or worse?
- Are there any stressors in your life?

Enquire About
- Mood
- Sleep
- Appetite
- Energy levels
- Concentration
- Auditory hallucinations
- Visual hallucinations
- Paranoid, persecutory and grandiose delusions

Risk Assessment
- Overspending
- Increased interest in sex
- Fire risk
- Driving risk
- Suicidal thoughts
- Thoughts of harming others [5]

Substance and Alcohol Misuse
- May I ask if you take alcohol in excess?
- May I ask if you take any recreational drugs?

Psychiatric History

Has he seen a psychiatrist in the past?

Medical History

Does he have any medical problems?

Medication and Compliance
- Do you take any regular medication?
- Any recent changes in dose of medication [6]?

Mild Cognitive Impairment

Scenario

78-year-old Henrietta Gilbert has been having a few memory issues. A detailed history and cognitive tests including mini-mental state examination have been completed. She appears to have mild cognitive impairment.

Task

Explain her condition and answer her queries.

Approach

Hello, I am Dr. ____. I understand you are here to discuss the outcome of the tests that you have done. Is that right?

- Mild cognitive impairment is the stage in between the expected memory decline of normal ageing and the more pronounced decline of dementia.
- It can involve problems with memory, language, thinking and decision-making.
- Information is gathered from the individual and family; we also complete numerous tests and assessments.
- The basic activities of daily living are managed well by the individual.
- There is minimal disruption in more complex functions.
- Many people with mild cognitive impairment do not develop dementia; however, there is an increased risk of individuals going on to develop dementia in the future.
- There is approximately a 10% chance each year of mild cognitive impairment progressing to dementia.
- It is important to follow a healthy diet that is low in saturated fats with plenty of fruits and vegetables, stop smoking and abstain from alcohol.
- Engage in regular exercise of at least 30 min, 5 days a week.
- Ensure adequate stimulation for the brain by reading, doing crossword puzzles or sudoku and regular social interactions with friends and family.
- Risk factors for developing dementia—female gender, Down's syndrome, presence of a protein called apolipoprotein E, history of depression and less than 8 years of education [7].
- Leaflets.

Behavioural and Psychological Symptoms of Dementia

Scenario

87-year-old David Johnson has a diagnosis of Alzheimer's dementia and resides in a care home. He has been displaying aggressive behaviour recently, necessitating the use of olanzapine. His son has come to visit him and would like to speak to you.

Task

Speak to his son Paul and answer his questions.

Approach

I am Dr. ___. I am a psychiatrist. I understand you have a few questions.

Q1. I spoke to the nursing staff and understand my father has been aggressive; I am surprised as this is completely unlike him. Why do you think he is behaving in this manner?

A1. When a person has dementia, the behaviour can change sometimes. This is called behavioural and psychological symptoms of dementia.

Q2. I also understand he has been started on a medication called olanzapine.

A2. The National Institute for Health and Care Excellence guidelines recommend the use of an antipsychotic to make the situation safe for the individual and the people around him.

Q3. What are the side effects of this medication?

A3. Feeling more sleepy, changes in blood pressure and an increased risk of stroke.

Q4. That sounds concerning.

A4. Please allow me to reassure you that choice of medication is based on individual benefit-risk analysis. The medication will be kept under regular review and used at the lowest possible dose and for the shortest duration of time.

Q5. What other strategies do you use to help my father?

A5. Optimisation of the environment to be natural home-like and comfortable.

Using family pictures and paintings that are familiar to him.

Engaging the individual in meaningful activities and using structured routines that offer optimal stimulation to avoid boredom.

Other forms of therapy like aromatherapy, music therapy and reminiscence therapy.

We do a thorough assessment to look for health difficulties like depression or anxiety.

We also look for physical health issues like pain, constipation and infections [8].

Station-Specific Points

Be reassuring in your approach and answer queries in jargon-free language.

References

1. National Institute for Health and Care Excellence. Dementia: assessment, management and support for people living with dementia and their carers NICE guideline [NG97]. 2018. https://www.nice.org.uk/guidance/ng97/chapter/recommendations#pharmacological-interventions-for-dementia. Accessed 20 June.
2. Kales HC, Gitlin LN, Lyketsos CG. Assessment and management of behavioural and psychological symptoms of dementia. BMJ. 2015;350:h369.

3. World Health Organization. Dementia (BlockL2-6D8). 6D81 Vascular dementia. ICD-11 International Classification of Diseases—mortality and morbidity statistics. 11th revision ed. World Health Organization; 2018. p. 187.

4. Taylor DM, Barnes T, Young A. Chapter 6. Prescribing in older people. Dementia with Lewy bodies. The Maudsley prescribing guidelines in psychiatry. 14th ed. Wiley Blackwell; 2021. p. 624.

5. Casey P, Kelly B. Fish's clinical psychopathology signs and symptoms in psychiatry. 3rd ed. The Royal College of Psychiatrists; 2016.

6. Semple D, Smyth R. Chapter 2. Psychiatric assessment. History. Mental state examination. Oxford Handbook of Psychiatry. 3rd ed. Oxford University Press; 2017. p. 42–44.

7. Knopman DS, Petersen RC. Mild cognitive impairment and mild dementia: a clinical perspective. Mayo Clin Proc. 2014;89(10):1452.

8. Cerejeira J, Lagarto L, Mukaetova-Ladinska EB. Behavioural and psychological symptoms of dementia. Front Neurol. 2012;3:73. https://doi.org/10.3389/fneur.2012.00073.

Child and Adolescent Psychiatry and Learning Disability

Autism Spectrum Disorder

Scenario

10-year-old Jack Roberts has been referred by the GP since he has been having some difficulties at school. The GP is querying a diagnosis of autism spectrum disorder.

Task

Take a history from his mother Mrs. Roberts to establish the diagnosis.

Approach

Hello, I am Dr. _____. I am a psychiatrist. I understand Jack is having some difficulties at school. Please could you tell me more?

History of Presenting Complaint

Impaired Social Interaction
- Does he have any close friends?
- Does he find it difficult to make or keep friends?
- How does he feel about socialising in groups?

All names and scenarios mentioned in this book are fictitious. Any resemblance to actual individuals or backgrounds is entirely conincidental.

© The Author(s), under exclusive license to Springer Nature Switzerland AG 2023
N. Sivaswamy, *Prepare for the MRCPsych CASC Exam*,
https://doi.org/10.1007/978-3-031-31019-5_3

- Does he have difficulty maintaining eye contact when speaking to someone?
- Is he able to understand the feelings and emotions of others—for example, if someone was upset, would he know how to comfort them?

Impaired Communication
- Does he have difficulty understanding people during social interactions?
- Have there been occasions when he felt that others did not understand him?
- Does he take things people say literally?
- Can he understand if someone says a joke?

Restricted Stereotyped Interests and Behaviours
- Does he have any specific interests—what is it you are interested in?
- Does he do certain things repeatedly?
- Do certain things have to be in a specific way—routines or rituals?
- How would he cope with change in routines?

Developmental History
- Milestones
- Playing with other children
- Sharing toys
- Lining up toys
- Sensory issues—sensitive to noise and certain textures of clothing/food
- Repetitive movements—hand flapping, rocking and spinning [1]

Impact and Coping
This sounds really difficult for you. How has this impacted on you and how are you coping?

Substance and Alcohol Misuse
May I ask if he takes any alcohol or recreational drugs?

Psychiatric History
Has he seen a psychiatrist in the past?

Medical History
Any medical issues?
   Does he take any regular medication?

Family History
Anyone in the family with mental health issues?

Brief Mental State Examination
Ask about mood, sleep, appetite, anhedonia, generalised anxiety, and auditory and visual hallucinations.

Risk Assessment
Suicidal thoughts or plans, thoughts of harming others and deliberate self-harm [2]

Attention Deficit Hyperactivity Disorder

Scenario

8-year-old Graeme Souter has been seen by the GP due to concerns raised by his mother regarding overactivity. The GP has referred to child psychiatric services to assess for attention deficit hyperactivity disorder.

Task

Take a history from his mother Mrs. Souter to establish the diagnosis.

Approach

Hello, I am Dr. ____. I am a psychiatrist. I understand you have some concerns about Graeme. Please could you tell me more?

Concentration
- Does he have difficulty paying attention to tasks?
- Does he make careless mistakes frequently?
- Does he struggle to concentrate on tasks?
- Do you find him easily distracted?
- Does he have trouble following a set of instructions?

Hyperactivity
- Is he able to wait for his turn?
- Does he have trouble sitting still?
- Does he talk too much?
- Does he frequently interrupt others?

Impulsive
- Do you think he behaves impulsively at times?
- Does he put himself in dangerous situations at times due to his impulsive behaviours?
- How is his sense of road safety?

  School—any issues with listening to his teachers?
  Home—is he able to sit with the family for mealtimes?

Developmental History
- Milestones
- Playing with other children [3]

Impact and Coping
This sounds really difficult for you. How has this impacted on you and how are you coping?

Substance and Alcohol Misuse
May I ask if he takes any alcohol or recreational drugs?

Psychiatric History
Has he seen a psychiatrist in the past?

Medical History
Any medical issues?

Family History
Anyone in the family with mental health issues?

Brief Mental State Examination
Ask about mood, sleep, appetite, anhedonia, generalised anxiety, and auditory and visual hallucinations.

Risk Assessment
Suicidal thoughts or plans, thoughts of harming others and deliberate self-harm [2]

Attention Deficit Hyperactivity Disorder Management

Scenario

7-year-old Paul Gables has been recently diagnosed with attention deficit hyperactivity disorder . His mother is waiting to speak to you to discuss management options for his condition.

Task

Discuss the management of attention deficit hyperactivity disorder.

Approach

Hello, I am Dr. _____. I am a psychiatrist. I understand Paul has been recently diagnosed with ADHD, and we are here to speak about treatment options.

Explain Attention Deficit Hyperactivity Disorder
- Do you have a reasonable understanding of attention deficit hyperactivity disorder or would you like me to briefly discuss that?

- Attention deficit hyperactivity disorder consists of three main symptoms—hyperactivity, impulsivity and poor concentration with easy distractibility.
- These behaviours are normal in children; however, in attention deficit hyperactivity disorder, these characteristics are exaggerated when compared to other children of the same age.
- Diagnosis is made by paediatricians or child psychiatrists based on information from teachers, parents and questionnaires.

Aetiology
- It can run in families.
- It can be related to problems during the pregnancy or birth of the child.
- It can be difficult to identify a particular cause [3].

Management
1. The National Institute for Health and Care Excellence guidelines recommend the use of a medication called methylphenidate.
2. It is a stimulant that affects part of the brain involved with attention and makes the child more focused.
3. Side effects—tummy aches, feeling sick, headaches, reduced appetite, staying awake later than usual at night and not growing as well as they should be.
4. We monitor for these side effects by regular checks of height, weight and blood pressure.
5. We can consider medication-free weekends, that is, only medicating the child during school days.
6. Behavioural management.
    - Using a reward system to encourage positive behaviours.
    - Liaise with school to provide specialised support including remedial training for teachers.
7. Psychoeducation.
8. Social interventions.
9. Parenting groups.
10. Social skill training to help the child manage their emotions better and improve confidence.

Additional Points
- There is no blood test to confirm the diagnosis.
- There is no need for a special diet; however, you might consider avoiding caffeine and foods high in sugar/preservatives if you find this helpful [4].

Childhood Maltreatment Management

Scenario

15-year-old Betty Archibald was admitted to the paediatric assessment unit following an overdose of 12 tablets of paracetamol. She is medically fit for discharge, and a psychiatric review has been requested prior to discharge. You are the psychiatrist on-call, and during your assessment, Betty revealed that she has been sexually assaulted by her stepfather on two occasions. She has not confided this to anyone previously and felt unable to tell her mother about this.

Task

Discuss the management of this patient with the staff nurse Stephanie on paediatric assessment unit.

Approach

Hello, I am Dr. _____. I am a psychiatrist. I was asked to review Betty following the overdose. During our conversation, she alleged that she has been sexually assaulted on two occasions by her stepfather.

Management
1. Due to the serious nature of the allegation, I terminated the assessment at this time.
2. I have asked a staff member to sit with Betty while I discussed a management plan with yourself.
3. I have informed Betty about the necessity to break confidentiality and share information with other agencies and colleagues.
4. I will inform the child protection officer.
5. Discuss with the hospital lead consultant for child protection concerns.
6. I will contact social services and refer her to them.
7. I will inform her mother.
8. She needs to remain in hospital for ongoing assessment of mental state including risk assessment.
9. We also need to identify potential risk to any siblings at home.
10. I would advise she be kept on one-to-one observation.
11. Her stepfather should not be allowed to see her to avoid causing her further distress.
12. Hospital security or the police can be involved if necessary.
13. I will convene an urgent multidisciplinary team meeting to make sure that all services can work together to support this child.
14. Long-term management—counselling and talking therapy [5].

Station-Specific Points

- The staff member may be dealing with their ward issues and may have their own bed pressures to manage.

- Discuss the management in a transparent and respectful manner.
- Emphasise the duty of care toward the child and that their safety is paramount.

Down's Syndrome with Dementia

Scenario

49-year-old Ewen Dreyfus has a diagnosis of Down's syndrome with moderate learning disability and has been referred by the GP with concerns that he is developing dementia.

Task

Take a collateral history from his mother, Mrs. Dreyfus.

Approach

Hello, I am Dr. ___. I am a psychiatrist. I understand you have some concerns about Ewen. Please could you tell me more?

History of Presenting Complaint
- When did you start noticing problems?
- Did it start gradually or suddenly?
- How has it progressed?

Does he
- Remember events from a few years ago
- Have difficulty recognising objects
- Have word finding difficulties
- Understand when someone speaks to him
- Have difficulty in doing things he used to be able to previously do
- Has he been more irritable recently?
- Has he had any aggressive episodes?

Brief Mental State Examination
Ask about mood, sleep, appetite, anhedonia, social withdrawal, generalised anxiety, and auditory and visual hallucinations.

Physical Problems
- Has there been a change in his gait or the way he walks?
- Has he been incontinent?
- Any abnormal movements of his body?
- Thyroid problems?

Psychiatric History
Has he seen a psychiatrist in the past?

Medical History and Medication
- Does he have any medical problems?
- Is he on medication?
- Does he take it regularly as prescribed?
- Have there been any changes in his medication?

Alcohol or Substance Misuse
- Does he take alcohol in excess?
- Does he take recreational drugs?

Family History
Anyone in the family with physical or mental health issues?

Risk Assessment
- Suicidal thoughts or plans
- Falls
- Wandering
- Aggression
- Driving risk
- Financial mismanagement
- Carers' strain [6]

Self-injurious Behaviours in Learning Disability

Scenario

20-year-old Douglas Slate has a diagnosis of severe learning disability. He has recently started engaging in self-injurious behaviour like biting and head banging. His mother is very concerned about his behaviour.

Task

Take a history from his mother Mrs. Slate, and identify possible aetiological factors.

Approach

Hello, I am Dr. ___. I understand you have some concerns about your son. Would you like to tell me more?

History of Presenting Complaint
- When did this first start?
- What was happening in his life around that time?
- Did it start suddenly or gradually?
- How has it progressed?
- Is there anything that makes these behaviours better or worse?
- Has anything like this happened before?

Any recent changes in
- Carers
- Routines
- Environment
- Hearing or vision
- Gait

Have you noticed
- Weakness of his hands and legs
- Any abnormal movements
- Any incontinence
- Any communication difficulties
- Any stressful events in his life

Substance and Alcohol Misuse
- May I ask if he takes alcohol in excess?
- May I ask if he takes any recreational drugs?

Psychiatric History
Has he seen a psychiatrist in the past?

Medical History
Any medical problems like

- Stroke
- High blood pressure
- Diabetes
- Epilepsy
- Infections
- Head injury
- Constipation

Medication and Compliance
- Is he on any regular medication?
- Does he take this medication as prescribed?
- Any recent changes in medication?

Family History
Anyone in the family with any mental or physical health issues?

Brief Mental State Examination

Enquire about mood, sleep, appetite, anhedonia, generalised anxiety, auditory/visual hallucinations and thought disorder.

Risk

- Has he expressed any suicidal thoughts?
- Has he self-harmed by cutting or any other means?
- Has he been aggressive?
- Enquire about carer strain.
- Is there any chance he might have been abused in any way at all [7]?

Station-Specific Points

Explore recent changes in carers, routines and environment.

Paediatric Overdose Assessment

Scenario

15-year-old Isla Boris has been admitted to A&E following an overdose of paracetamol tablets.

Task

Assess the circumstances of the overdose, and decide if she can be discharged to her parents' care or needs to remain in hospital.

Approach

Hello, I am Dr. ___. I am a psychiatrist. I understand you have taken an overdose.

- Why did you take the overdose?
- Could you please tell me how many tablets you took?
- Did you take all the tablets in one go or over a period of time?
- Where did you get the tablets?
- Did you plan this or was it impulsive?
- Where were you when you took the overdose?
- Did you wait for a time when there would be no one in the house to take the overdose?
- Did you lock the door?
- Did you tell anyone before you took the overdose?
- Did you send any emails or messages after you took the overdose?

- Did you write any goodbye letters or suicide notes?
- How did you come to the hospital?
- Why did you take the overdose?

Mental State Examination
- Mood
- Sleep
- Appetite
- Are you still able to enjoy the things you previously enjoyed?
- Do you see things when there is no one around you?
- Do you hear voices when there is no one around you?

Substance and Alcohol Misuse
- May I ask if you take alcohol?
- May I ask if you take any recreational drugs?

Psychiatric History
Have you seen a psychiatrist in the past?

Family History
Anyone in the family with any mental or physical health issues?

Medication and Compliance
Do you take any regular medication?

Risk
- What was your intent when taking the overdose?
- Do you regret taking the overdose?
- Do you have thoughts of ending your life now?
- How often do you have these thoughts?
- How intense are they?
- When they do occur, how long do they last?
- Have you ever tried to end your life previously?
- Do you deliberately self-harm by any means?

Social History
- How is your relationship with your family?
- Any friends who can offer support?
- Do you have any stressors at home or school—bullying—relationships [8]?

Station-Specific Points

Clearly state if she can go home or needs to remain in hospital.

Learning Disability and Pregnancy

Scenario

Mrs. Catherine Novak has come to speak to you regarding her concerns about her 19-year-old son Tom Novak who has a diagnosis of moderate learning disability. He lives with his girlfriend who also has learning difficulties, and they have recently found out that she is 7 weeks pregnant.

Task

Speak to Mrs. Novak and answer her questions.

Approach

Hello, I am Dr. ___ and I am a psychiatrist. I understand you are having some concerns about your son Tom.

Sterilisation
- Sterilisation is not considered an option. All people including those with learning disability have the same rights.
- Sterilisation is only performed for medical reasons that are in the best interests of the individual.
- Forced sterilisation is against the law.
- Informed consent of the individual is always required.
- Another person cannot give consent on the individual's behalf.

Developmental History
- Was the pregnancy planned or unplanned?
- Any complications during pregnancy?
- Any complications during delivery?
- Any problems with the baby after his birth?
- Any delays in crawling and walking?
- Any delays in his speech or language?
- When was the diagnosis of learning disability made?

Family History
Anyone in the family with similar problems as Tom?

Additional Points
- Not all cases of learning disability are passed from one generation to the next.
- The reasons can be multifactorial with no clear cause.
- Pregnancy ultrasound scans will screen for any obvious abnormalities.

Support

- Social work will offer a parenting assessment and support as needed if appropriate.
- You can choose to be involved as much or as little as you would like to be with the baby [9].

References

1. World Health Organization. Neurodevelopmental disorders (BlockL1-6A0). 6A02 Autism spectrum disorder. ICD-11 International Classification of Diseases—mortality and morbidity statistics. 11th revision ed. World Health Organization; 2018. p. 7.
2. Semple D, Smyth R. Chapter 2. Psychiatric assessment. History. Mental state examination. Oxford handbook of psychiatry. 3rd ed. Oxford University Press; 2017. p. 42–44.
3. World Health Organization. Neurodevelopmental disorders (BlockL1-6A0). 6A05 Attention deficit hyperactivity disorder. ICD-11 International Classification of Diseases—mortality and morbidity statistics. 11th revision ed. World Health Organization; 2018. p. 11.
4. National Institute for Health and Care Excellence. Management of attention deficit hyperactivity disorder (ADHD). https://cks.nice.org.uk/topics/attention-deficit-hyperactivity-disorder/management/management/. Accessed October 2022.
5. National Institute for Health and Care Excellence. Managing a child or young person where maltreatment is suspected or considered. 2019. https://cks.nice.org.uk/topics/child-maltreatment-recognition-management/management/managing-a-child-or-young-person-where-maltreatment-is-suspected-or-considered/. Accessed January.
6. Semple D, Smyth R. Chapter 18. Down's syndrome. Dementia in Down's syndrome. Oxford handbook of psychiatry. 3rd ed. Oxford University Press; 2017. p. 745.
7. National Institute for Health and Care Excellence. Challenging behaviour and learning disabilities: prevention and interventions for people with learning disabilities whose behaviour challenges. 2014; NICE Guideline for consultation.
8. Semple D, Smyth R. Liaison psychiatry. Parasuicide assessment. Oxford handbook of psychiatry. 3rd ed. Oxford University Press; 2017. p. 784.
9. Stansfield A, Holland A, Clare I. The sterilisation of people with intellectual disabilities in England and Wales during the period 1988 to 1999. J Intellect Disabil Res. 2007, 51(Pt 8):569–79.

Substance and Alcohol Misuse

Alcohol Dependence

Scenario

32-year-old Tom Wallace has been to see his GP today as his partner is concerned regarding his alcohol use. The GP has referred him to the alcohol misuse service for an outpatient appointment.

Task

Take a history of alcohol dependence.

Approach

Hello, I am Dr. _____. I am a psychiatrist. I understand you have been having some difficulties. I am sorry to hear that. Please could you tell me more?

History of Presenting Complaint
- What do you drink?
- How much do you drink in a day?
- Please talk me through a typical day including your alcohol use.

© The Author(s), under exclusive license to Springer Nature Switzerland AG 2023
N. Sivaswamy, *Prepare for the MRCPsych CASC Exam,*
https://doi.org/10.1007/978-3-031-31019-5_4

Elicit the Core Symptoms of Alcohol Dependence

- Do you crave for a drink sometimes?
- Do you neglect any other activities that make you happy so you can drink?
- Do you drink first thing in the morning?
- Do you find you have to drink more to achieve the same effect?

Impact

This sounds really difficult for you. How has this impacted on your

- Relationships
- Work—ask about late days and absences
- Driving—driving under the influence of alcohol
- Finances
- Health—medical problems like ulcers, fits, falls and head injury

May I ask if you take any recreational drugs?

Past History

- When did you first start drinking?
- What did you drink?
- How did you progress to current levels?
- Did you start drinking due to peer pressure or your own choice?
- Have you ever tried not to drink?
- What happens when you do not drink—sweating, shakiness, headaches and feeling sick?
- Have you ever had fits?
- Have you ever had a detox as an outpatient or inpatient?
- What is your longest period of abstinence?
- What made you start drinking again [1]?

Past Psychiatric History

Have you seen a psychiatrist in the past?

Family History

Anyone in the family with any mental or physical health issues?

Medication and Compliance

Do you take any regular medication?
    Do you take the medication as prescribed?

Brief Mental State Examination

Ask about mood, sleep, appetite, anhedonia, generalised anxiety, and auditory and visual hallucinations.

Risk Assessment

Suicidal thoughts or plans, thoughts of harming others and deliberate self-harm

Motivation to Change
- Do you think you have a problem with alcohol use?
- What would you like to happen [1]?

Opiate Dependence

Scenario

32-year-old Jasper Newman has a problem with opiate use.

Task

Take a history of opiate dependence.

Approach

Hello, I am Dr. ____. I am a psychiatrist. I understand you have been having some difficulties. I am sorry to hear that. Please could you tell me more?

History of Presenting Complaint
- What drugs do you use?
- Have you ever used any other drugs—cannabis, cocaine and amphetamines?
- What are you using now?
- How often do you use this?
- How much do you take in a day?
- Have you ever used more than one drug at the same time?
- How much money do you spend in a day or week on drugs?
- How do you finance your drug use?
- What is your preferred route for drug use—oral, smoking and injected?

  If injected
- What sites do you use for injecting?
- Have you ever shared needles?
- Are you familiar with the needle exchange programme?

Elicit the Core Symptoms of Opiate Dependence
- Do you crave for drugs sometimes?
- Do you find you have to take more amount to achieve the same effect?
- If you do not take drugs, do you experience withdrawal effects?

Impact
This sounds really difficult for you. How has this impacted on your

- Relationships
- Work—ask about late days and absences

- Driving—driving under the influence of drugs
- Finances
- Health—medical problems
  May I ask if you use alcohol in excess?

Complications of Drug Use

Ask about
- Screening for hepatitis B, hepatitis C, HIV
- Abscess
- Accidents
- Falls
- Head injury

Past History
- When did you first start using drugs?
- Did you start taking drugs due to peer pressure or your own choice?
- What was the first drug you took?
- How did you progress to current levels?
- Have you ever had any treatment for the drug problem?
- Have you ever been in hospital for your drug issues?
- Have you ever had any periods of abstinence?
- Why did you start using again?

Past Psychiatric History
Have you seen a psychiatrist in the past?

Family History
Anyone in the family with any mental or physical health issues?

Medication and Compliance
- Do you take any regular medication?
- Do you take the medication as prescribed?

Brief Mental State Examination
Ask about mood, sleep, appetite, anhedonia, generalised anxiety, and auditory and visual hallucinations.

Risk Assessment
Suicidal thoughts or plans, thoughts of harming others and deliberate self-harm

Motivation to Change
- Do you think you have a problem with drug use?
- What would you like to happen [2]?

Complications of Alcohol Use

Scenario

43-year-old Adrian Patters has been diagnosed with alcohol abuse.

Task

Assess the impact of alcohol abuse on his life.

Approach

Hello, I am Dr. ____. I am a psychiatrist. I would like to speak to you today to understand the impact alcohol use has had on your life.

History of Presenting Complaint
- What do you drink?
- How much do you drink in a day?
- Please talk me through a typical day including your alcohol use.

Impact

Relationship Difficulties
- Arguments
- Agitation
- Physical aggression

Work Issues
- Lateness
- Absences
- Drinking at work
- Warnings about poor performance

Police Issues
- Driving under the influence of alcohol
- Drunk and disorderly behaviour
- Damage to public property
- Charges
- Convictions

Financial Problems
- Debts

Social Issues
- Breakdown of relationships
- Loss of friends

- Social isolation

Physical Health Problems
- Ulcers
- Liver disease
- Falls
- Head injury
- Fits

Brief Mental State Examination

Ask about mood, sleep, appetite, anhedonia, generalised anxiety, and auditory and visual hallucinations.

Risk Assessment

Suicidal thoughts or plans, thoughts of harming others and deliberate self-harm [3]

Alcohol Dependence with Anxiety

Scenario

37-year-old Anne Mathers has been to see his GP today as she has been increasingly anxious at work. Her husband has also informed the GP he is concerned about her alcohol use.

Task

Take a history to ascertain her difficulties.

Approach

Hello, I am Dr. _____. I am a psychiatrist. I understand you have been having some difficulties. I am sorry to hear that. Please could you tell me more?

History of Presenting Complaint
- May I ask what difficulties you are experiencing?
- Do you feel you get anxious at times?
- When did this all first start?
- What was happening in your life at that time?
- How has this progressed?
- What kind of things make you anxious?
- When you do feel anxious, how long does this feeling last?
- How often in the course of a day can you feel this way?
- How do you feel between episodes?
- Anything that makes these feelings better or worse?

- Avoidance: Do you try to avoid things that might make you anxious?
- Anticipatory anxiety: Do you worry about when the next episode may occur?
- Are there any stressors in your life?
- How would you describe your personality?

Elicit the Symptoms Associated with Anxiety
- When you feel anxious, what kind of things do you experience in your body—heart racing, shortness of breath, sweating and dry mouth?
- And when you feel this way, what thoughts run through your mind—do you worry something awful will happen or do you worry about losing control?

Substance/Alcohol Misuse
- May I ask if you take any recreational drugs?
- May I ask if you take alcohol in excess?
- What do you drink?
- How much do you drink in a day?
- Please talk me through a typical day including your alcohol use.

Elicit the Core Symptoms of Alcohol Dependence
- Do you crave for a drink sometimes?
- Do you neglect any other activities that make you happy so you can drink?
- Do you drink first thing in the morning?
- Do you find you have to drink more to achieve the same effect?

Impact and Coping
This sounds difficult for you. How has this impacted on your

- Relationships
- Work—ask about late days and absences
- Driving—driving under the influence of alcohol
- Finances
- Health—medical problems like ulcers

Past History
- When did you first start drinking?
- What did you drink?
- How did you progress to current levels?
- Have you ever tried not to drink?
- What happens when you do not drink—sweating, shakiness, headaches and feeling sick?
- Have you ever had fits?

Past Psychiatric History
Have you seen a psychiatrist in the past?

Family History
Anyone in the family with any mental or physical health issues?

Medication and Compliance
- Do you take any regular medication?
- Do you take the medication as prescribed?

Brief Mental State Examination
Ask about mood, sleep, appetite, anhedonia, and auditory and visual hallucinations.

Risk Assessment
Suicidal thoughts or plans, thoughts of harming others and deliberate self-harm [4]

Alcoholic Hallucinosis

Scenario

44-year-old Patrick Alexander has been to see his GP today as he has been hearing voices for the last 2 days.

Task

Take a history of his problems to arrive at a provisional diagnosis.

Approach

Hello, I am Dr. _____. I am a psychiatrist. I understand you have been having some difficulties. I am sorry to hear that. Please could you tell me more?

- When did you first start hearing these voices?
- Have you experienced anything similar in the past?
- How often do you hear them?
- Is there anything that makes these voices better or worse?
- How many voices do you hear?
- Do they talk to you directly?
- Do they talk among themselves about you?
- What do they say?
- Do they ask you to harm yourself or others?
- Are the voices inside your head or from outside?

Impact and Coping
This sounds really difficult for you. How has this impacted on your

- Relationships
- Work
- Driving

Substance and Alcohol Misuse
- May I ask if you take any recreational drugs?
- May I ask if you drink any alcohol at all?
- What do you drink?
- How much do you drink in a day?
- Please talk me through a typical day including your alcohol use.

Additional Questions
- When did you stop drinking?
- Did you stop drinking gradually or suddenly?
- Have you experienced any sweating, shakiness, headaches and fits?
- Did you start hearing the voices after you stopped drinking?
- How long after you stopped drinking did you start hearing the voices?

Past Psychiatric History
Have you seen a psychiatrist in the past?

Family History
Anyone in the family with any mental or physical health issues?

Medication and Compliance
- Do you take any regular medication?
- Do you take the medication as prescribed?

Brief Mental State Examination
Ask about mood, sleep, appetite, anhedonia, generalised anxiety and visual hallucinations.

Risk Assessment
Suicidal thoughts or plans, thoughts of harming others and deliberate self-harm.

Explain the Diagnosis
The most likely diagnosis appears to be alcoholic hallucinosis. This is a complication of alcohol withdrawal that occurs 12–24 h after the last drink and presents as hearing voices that are threatening or accusatory [5].

GHB Dependence

Scenario

25-year-old Carter Hill collapsed at a party and was brought to hospital by his friends who informed he used GHB during the party.

Task

Take a history of GHB use.

Approach

Hello, I am Dr. _____. I am a psychiatrist. I understand you collapsed while attending a party. Please could you tell me more?

History of Presenting Circumstances
- What were you doing at the party when you collapsed?
- May I ask if you used any drugs like GHB at the party?
- How often do you use this?
- How much do you take in a day?
- How much did you take at the party?
- Was that more than you usually take?
- Why did you take more than your usual amount of the drug? What was your intention?
- Have you ever used more than one drug at the same time?
- How much money do you spend in a day or week on drugs?
- How do you finance your drug use?
- What is your preferred route for drug use—oral, smoking and injected? If injected
- What sites do you use for injecting?
- Have you ever shared needles?
- Have you ever heard of the needle exchange programme? Have you ever used any other drugs—cannabis, cocaine and amphetamines?

Elicit the Core Symptoms of Drug Dependence
- Do you crave for drugs sometimes?
- Do you find you have to take more amount to achieve the same effect?
- If you do not take drugs, do you experience withdrawal effects?

Impact
This sounds really difficult for you. How has this impacted on your

- Relationships
- Work—ask about late days and absences
- Driving—driving under the influence of drugs
- Finances
- Health—medical problems

  May I ask if you use alcohol in excess?

Additional Questions
- Have you ever had any treatment for drug-related issues?
- Have you ever been in hospital for drug-related issues?

- Have you ever had any periods of abstinence?
- Why did you start using again?

Complications of Drug Use
- Ask about screening for hepatitis B, hepatitis C and HIV.
- Abscess, accidents, falls and head injury.
- Have you previously had any drug overdoses?

Past History
- When did you first start using drugs?
- What was the first drug you took?
- How did you progress to current levels?

Past Psychiatric History
Have you seen a psychiatrist in the past?

Family History
Anyone in the family with any mental or physical health issues?

Medication and Compliance
- Do you take any regular medication?
- Do you take the medication as prescribed?

Brief Mental State Examination
Ask about mood, sleep, appetite, anhedonia, generalised anxiety, and auditory and visual hallucinations.

Risk Assessment
Suicidal thoughts or plans, thoughts of harming others and deliberate self-harm.

Motivation to Change
- Do you think you have a problem with drug use?
- What would you like to happen [6]?

Delirium Tremens Management

Scenario

52-year-old Timothy Sutton was admitted to the orthopaedic ward 3 days ago after a fall and sustained a hip fracture, which has since been operated on by the orthopaedic surgeons. In the last 24 h, he has been presenting with hallucinations, suspicious of the nurses on the ward and confused. You have taken a collateral history from his daughter who says that Timothy has been a heavy drinker for many years.

Task

Speak to the staff nurse Malcom on the orthopaedic ward, explain the diagnosis, discuss the management and answer his questions.

Approach

I am Dr. ___. I am a psychiatrist.

- Given that he is presenting with altered consciousness and hallucinations, last drink was prior to admission 3 days ago and the collateral history from his daughter confirms that he is a heavy drinker, the most likely diagnosis appears to be delirium tremens.
- It is a life-threatening medical condition requiring emergency treatment that presents as a toxic confusional state occurring when alcohol withdrawal symptoms are severe and usually manifests 72–96 h after the last drink.
- Typical symptoms are confusion, hallucinations and tremors.

Management
1. He needs to be managed in a medical ward as this is a medical emergency.
2. He requires close monitoring with staff trained to manage acute medical illness.
3. Monitoring of blood pressure, pulse, temperature and respiratory rate.
4. Optimisation of environment by ensuring that he is nursed in a quiet well-lit room with consistent nursing support with frequent reorientation.
5. Detoxification with chlordiazepoxide in a reducing regime.
6. Pabrinex injections intravenously administered three times a day to prevent Wernicke's encephalopathy.
7. Oral thiamine 100 mg three times a day.
8. He requires close monitoring for withdrawal seizures and Wernicke's encephalopathy.
9. Antipsychotics are used with extreme caution as they reduce the seizure threshold, thereby increasing the risk of seizures.
10. If the patient tries to leave, he can be held in hospital as assessment and treatment are in the patient's best interest; however, it is important to use the least restrictive methods.
11. They can be assessed for detention under the Mental Health Act if required.
12. Long term—referral to the alcohol liaison service and psychoeducation [7].

Alcohol Use and Impact on Mood

Scenario

32-year-old Mr. Jeffrey Radcliff was referred by the GP due to concerns about excessive alcohol use and low mood.

Task

Take a history of alcohol use and ascertain the impact on his mood.

Approach

Hello, I am Dr. _____. I am a psychiatrist. I understand you have been referred by the GP due to concerns about alcohol use and low mood. I am sorry to hear that. Please could you tell me more?

History of Presenting Complaint
- What do you drink?
- How much do you drink in a day?
- Please talk me through a typical day including your alcohol use.

Elicit the Core Symptoms of Alcohol Dependence
- Do you crave for a drink sometimes?
- Do you neglect any other activities that make you happy so you can drink?
- Do you drink first thing in the morning?
- Do you find you have to drink more to achieve the same effect?

Impact and Coping
This sounds really difficult for you. How has this impacted on your

- Relationships
- Work—ask about late days and absences
- Driving—driving under the influence of alcohol
- Finances
- Health—medical problems like ulcers
  May I ask if you take any recreational drugs?

Additional Questions
- Have you ever tried not to drink?
- What happens when you do not drink—sweating, shakiness, headaches and feeling sick?
- Have you ever had fits?
- Have you ever had a detox as an outpatient or inpatient?
- What is your longest period of abstinence?
- What made you start drinking again?

Past History
- When did you first start drinking?
- What did you drink?
- How did you progress to current levels?

Past Psychiatric History

Have you seen a psychiatrist in the past?

Family History

Anyone in the family with any mental or physical health issues?

Medication and Compliance

- Do you take any regular medication?
- Do you take the medication as prescribed?

Mental State Examination

Ask about mood, sleep, appetite, anhedonia, memory, concentration, motivation, self-esteem, feelings of guilt, generalised anxiety, auditory and visual hallucinations, thought disorder and delusions.

Risk Assessment

Suicidal thoughts or plans, thoughts of harming others and deliberate self-harm [8]

References

1. NICE clinical guidelines, no. 115. National Collaborating Centre for Mental Health (UK). Leicester (UK). Alcohol-use disorders: diagnosis, assessment and management of harmful drinking and alcohol dependence. The British Psychological Society and The Royal College of Psychiatrists; 2011.
2. Semple D, Smyth R. Substance misuse. Assessment of the drug user. Oxford handbook of psychiatry. 3rd ed. Oxford University Press; 2017. p. 592.
3. Semple D, Smyth R. Assessment of the patient with alcohol problems. Oxford handbook of psychiatry. 3rd ed. Oxford University Press; 2017. p. 552.
4. World Health Organization. 6C40.71 Alcohol-induced anxiety disorder. ICD-11 International Classification of Diseases—mortality and morbidity statistics. 11th ed. World Health Organization; 2018. p. 71.
5. World Health Organization. 6C40.60 Alcohol-induced psychotic disorder with hallucinations. ICD-11 International Classification of Diseases—mortality and morbidity statistics. 11th revision ed. World Health Organization; 2018. p. 70.
6. Taylor DM, Barnes T, Young A. GHB and GBL dependence. The Maudsley prescribing guidelines in psychiatry. 14th ed. Wiley Blackwell; 2021. p. 514.
7. Taylor DM, Barnes T, Young A. Alcohol withdrawal delirium—delirium tremens. The Maudsley prescribing guidelines in psychiatry. 14th ed. Wiley Blackwell; 2021. p. 472.
8. World Health Organization. Disorders due to substance use (BlockL2-6C4). 6C40.70 Alcohol-induced mood disorder. ICD-11 International Classification of Diseases—Mortality and Morbidity Statistics. 11th revision ed. World Health Organization; 2018. p. 71.

Conversion Disorder

Scenario

18-year-old Rachel Daniels presented with sudden paralysis of her lower limbs. All preliminary medical investigations including neurological examination are normal.

Task

Take a history, and identify any precipitating factors for her condition.

Approach

Hello, I am Dr. _____. I am a psychiatrist. I understand you have been having some difficulties. I am sorry to hear that. Please could you tell me more?

History of Presenting Complaint
- When did all this first start?
- What was happening in your life at that time?
- Any stressful life event, conflicts and physical health issues?
- Has anything like this happened before?
- Are there any triggers that make you think this way?
- Is there anything that makes these thoughts better or worse?

All names and scenarios mentioned in this book are fictitious. Any resemblance to actual individuals or backgrounds is entirely conincidental.

© The Author(s), under exclusive license to Springer Nature Switzerland AG 2023

N. Sivaswamy, *Prepare for the MRCPsych CASC Exam*, https://doi.org/10.1007/978-3-031-31019-5_5

- Any ongoing stressors in your life?
- Primary gain: Do you feel less worried or anxious at present?
- Secondary gain: Do you find yourself getting more attention?
- Do you find anything positive about your current situation [1]?

Impact and Coping

This sounds really difficult for you. How has this impacted on your

- Relationships
- Work

  With all this going on, how have you been coping?

- May I ask if you take alcohol in excess?
- May I ask if you take any recreational drugs?

Psychiatric History

Have you seen a psychiatrist in the past?

Family History

Anyone in the family with any mental or physical issues?

Medication and Compliance

- Do you have any medical problems?
- Do you take any regular medication?

Brief Mental State Examination

Ask about mood, sleep, appetite, anhedonia, generalised anxiety, auditory and visual hallucinations and insight.

Risk Assessment

Suicidal thoughts or plans, thoughts of harming others and deliberate self-harm [2]

Station-Specific Points

- Anticipate that the actor may not be forthcoming with information.
- Be empathic and build a good rapport.

Body Dysmorphic Disorder

Scenario

21-year-old May Burns is unhappy with her appearance and feels her eyes are set far apart.

Task

Take a history.

Approach

Hello, I am Dr. _____. I am a psychiatrist. I understand you have some concerns about your appearance. I am sorry to hear that. Please could you tell me more?

History of Presenting Complaint
- Please could you tell me what you are concerned about.
- Has anyone else noticed this?
- When did all this first start?
- What was happening in your life at that time?
- Has anything like this happened before?
- Any other part of your body you are unhappy about?
- Are there any triggers that make you think this way?
- Is there anything that makes these thoughts better or worse?
- Any ongoing stressors in your life?

Enquire About Time-Consuming Behaviours
- Repeated checking of appearance
- Frequent mirror gazing to check appearance
- Excessive camouflage to conceal the perceived flaw
- Grooming rituals [3]

Impact and Coping
This sounds really difficult for you. How has this impacted on your

- Relationships
- Work
- Social life—social withdrawal and lack of self-confidence

    With all this going on, how have you been coping?

- May I ask if you take alcohol in excess?
- May I ask if you take any recreational drugs at all?

Psychiatric History
Have you seen a psychiatrist in the past?

Family History
Anyone in the family with any mental or physical health issues?

Medication and Compliance
- Do you take any regular medication?
- Do you take the medication as prescribed?

Brief Mental State Examination

- Ask about mood, sleep, appetite, anhedonia, generalised anxiety, and auditory and visual hallucinations.
- Did this thought about your eyes occur out of the blue or following an unusual experience?
- How convinced are you?
- Could there be another explanation?
- Have you told anyone else? What did they say?

Risk Assessment

- Suicidal thoughts or plans.
- Thoughts of harming others.
- Deliberate self-harm.
- Driving: Have you ever had any accidents or problems with the police due to checking your appearance in the car mirrors?
- Have you made any attempts to fix your appearance yourself?
- Is there a chance you may try to alter your appearance yourself if you did not get the help you think you need [2]?

Station-Specific Points

Enquire about time-consuming behaviours.

Hypochondriasis

Scenario

36-year-old Samuel Finnie has been referred by the GP as he remains concerned about frequent headaches despite all investigations being normal. He believes that he has brain cancer.

Task

Take a history.

Approach

Hello, I am Dr. ____. I am a psychiatrist. I understand you have some concerns. Please could you tell me more?

History of Presenting Complaint
- Please could you tell me what you are concerned about? Elicit the specific concern.
- When did all this first start?
- What was happening in your life at that time?
- Has anything similar happened before?
- Any other medical issues in your body that you worry about?
- Are there any triggers that make you feel this way?
- Is there anything that makes this better or worse?
- Any ongoing stressors in your life?

Enquire About
- Information-seeking behaviours.

Have you been checking various sources like the internet or magazines to find more information about this?

- I understand you have had several investigations done; do you find that reassuring?
- How long before you feel the need to seek medical help again?

How much time do you spend worrying about this [4]?

Impact and Coping
This sounds really difficult for you. How has this impacted on your

- Relationships
- Work
- Social life

With all this going on, how have you been coping?

- May I ask if you take alcohol in excess?
- May I ask if you take any recreational drugs?

Psychiatric History
- Have you seen a psychiatrist in the past?

Family History
- Anyone in the family with any mental or physical health issues?

Childhood
- History of medical issues in family or self as a child, necessitating frequent hospital visits
- Excessive medical attention-seeking parents

Medication and Compliance
- Do you take any regular medication?

- Do you take the medication as prescribed?

Brief Mental State Examination
- Ask about mood, sleep, appetite, anhedonia, generalised anxiety, and auditory and visual hallucinations.
- Do you think you have an underlying issue that has been overlooked?
- What medical problem do you think you might have?

Risk Assessment
- Suicidal thoughts or plans, thoughts of harming others and deliberate self-harm.
- Have you made any attempts to fix your issues yourself [2]?

Station-Specific Points

- Explore the presence of information-seeking behaviours.
- Explore the presence of preoccupation and rumination.

Bodily Distress Disorder

Scenario

45-year-old Thomas Jackson has been referred by the GP since he has been concerned about pain in his back. All medical investigations have been normal.

Task

Take a history.

Approach

Hello, I am Dr. _____. I am a psychiatrist. I understand you have been having some concern regarding pain in your back. I am sorry to hear that. Please could you tell me more?

History of Presenting Complaint
- May I ask what concerns you have?
- When did this all start?
- What was happening in your life at that time?
- Are you concerned about anything else?

Elicit the Details of His Concerns

- Elicit a full description of the pain—onset, duration, progression, frequency and severity.
- Anything that makes the pain worse?
- Anything that makes the pain better?
- What have you done about the pain?
- How do you manage the pain?
- Medication requests: Have you repeatedly requested you be prescribed medication for the pain?
- What do you think is the reason for the pain?
- Do you think there is some underlying reason for the pain that has not been discovered so far?
- What have the doctors told you about your issues [5]?

Impact and Coping

This sounds really difficult for you. How has this impacted on your

- Relationships
- Work

  With all this going on, how have you been coping?

- May I ask if you take alcohol in excess?
- May I ask if you take any recreational drugs?

Psychiatric History

Have you seen a psychiatrist in the past?

Family History

Anyone in the family with any mental or physical health issues?

Medication and Compliance

Do you take any regular medication?

Brief Mental State Examination

- Ask about mood, sleep, appetite, anhedonia, generalised anxiety, and auditory and visual hallucinations.
- Did this pain start out of the blue or following an unusual experience?
- How convinced are you that you are having this problem?
- Could there be any other explanation?
- Have you told anyone else? What did they say?

Risk Assessment

- Suicidal thoughts or plans, thoughts of harming others and deliberate self-harm.
- Have you tried to manage the pain yourself?
- Do you think you might hurt yourself in an attempt to manage your pain [2]?

Station-Specific Points

Enquire about the risk of him trying to hurt himself in an effort to manage the pain.

Overdose Risk Assessment

Scenario

24-year-old Jenna Howard was admitted to A&E following an overdose of 30 paracetamol tablets. She is medically fit for discharge and is waiting to be reviewed by the psychiatrist.

Task

Take a history of the circumstances around the overdose.
    Perform a detailed risk assessment.

Approach

Hello, I am Dr. _____. I am a psychiatrist. I understand you were admitted to A&E following an overdose. I am sorry to hear that.

History of Presenting Complaint
- Please could you take me through the circumstances leading to the overdose?
- What were you doing just before you took the overdose?
- Where were you when you took the overdose?
- Did you make attempts to avoid being found—locking the door or wait till you were alone in the house?
- What did you take? Anything else?
- Did you believe you could end your life by doing this?
- Did you take any alcohol or recreational drugs at that time?
- How did you manage to find these many tablets?
- Was the overdose impulsive or planned?
- Did you send any emails, messages or phone family or friends to tell them about the overdose?
- Did you write a suicide note?
- Has anything similar happened before?
- Is there anything that makes this better or worse?
- Any ongoing stressors in your life?

Impact and Coping
This sounds really difficult for you. How has this impacted on your

- Relationships
- Work
  With all this going on, how have you been coping?
- May I ask if you take alcohol in excess?
- May I ask if you take any recreational drugs?

Psychiatric History
- Have you seen a psychiatrist in the past?

Family History
- Anyone in the family with any mental or physical health issues?

Social History
- Who do you live with at present?
- Do you have friends or family who are able to offer support?

Medication and Compliance
- Do you take any regular medication?
- Do you take the medication as prescribed?

Brief Mental State Examination
- Ask about mood, sleep, appetite, anhedonia, generalised anxiety, and auditory and visual hallucinations.

Risk Assessment
- Looking back on what has happened, how do you feel about it now?
- Do you regret having taken the overdose?
- Suicidal thoughts or plans: Do you have any suicidal thoughts? Do you have any specific plans?
- Previous suicidal attempts: Have you tried to end your life before? Enquire the details of these attempts.
- Do you harm yourself in other ways like cutting and burning?
- Do you have thoughts of harming anyone else?
- If we offer you further appointments with psychiatric services, would you attend?
- If we offer medication, would you take it as advised [6]?

Station-Specific Points

- Explore preparation, planning and precaution.
- Enquire about help-seeking behaviours.
- Take a detailed social history.

Dissociative Stupor

Scenario

19-year-old Bess Wooley was admitted to hospital after she collapsed while walking to university with her friends who called an ambulance. The friends informed that they were listening to the news on the radio while walking through the park on their way to the college. In hospital, all medical investigations and physical examination are normal. However, she is not speaking or moving despite being fully conscious. Her mother Mrs. Wooley is waiting to speak to you.

Task

Take a brief history from Mrs. Wooley.
    Explain the diagnosis and devise a management plan.

Approach

Hello, I am Dr. ___. I am a psychiatrist. I understand you have some concerns. Please could you tell me more?

History of Presenting Circumstances
- Please could you tell me how you came to know of your daughter being admitted to hospital?

  When she collapsed, did she have any

- Odd movements of her body
- Tongue biting
- Incontinence
- Head injury

  What was she doing when she collapsed?
  Any ongoing stressors in her life?

Substance and Alcohol Misuse
- May I ask if she takes alcohol in excess?
- May I ask if she takes any recreational drugs?

Psychiatric History
Has she seen a psychiatrist in the past?

Family History
Anyone in the family with any mental or physical issues?

Medication and Compliance

Does she take any regular medication?

Does she take the medication as prescribed?

Brief Mental State Examination

Ask about her mood, sleep, appetite, anhedonia, generalised anxiety, auditory and visual hallucinations and insight.

Risk Assessment

Suicidal thoughts or plans, thoughts of harming others and deliberate self-harm [2]

Explain the Diagnosis

- The most likely diagnosis appears to be dissociative stupor: Have you heard of this before?
- Dissociative stupor is a condition whereby when the person experiences an event that is mentally stressful, the body reacts by becoming unresponsive despite the individual being fully conscious.
- • All investigations show no physical cause for her current presentation.

Management

1. As she is not eating or drinking, she needs to remain in the medical ward.
2. Advise parents not to collude with the individual: it is important not to reinforce the sick role and encourage her to be independent.
3. Benzodiazepines like lorazepam will be tried first line.
4. Electroconvulsive therapy can be tried as the last resort if there are significant concerns for the individual's health.
5. Long term—psychological therapy to address the root cause of any stressors [7].

Traumatic Brain Injury

Scenario

36-year-old Jefferson Walker has experienced a change in his personality since his recent car accident.

Task

Take a history.

Approach

Hello, I am Dr. ___. I am a psychiatrist. I understand you have been having some difficulties. Would you like to tell me more?

Details of the Accident
- When did the accident occur?
- Did you have any physical injuries?
- Any head injuries?
- Loss of consciousness
- Vomiting
- Fits
- Headaches

Presenting Complaints
- Did your difficulties start suddenly or gradually?
- How have these difficulties progressed?
- Is there anything that makes your difficulties better or worse?

Personality Change
- Socially inappropriate behaviour
- Decreased social awareness

Behavioural Change
- Apathy
- Loss of spontaneity
- Loss of motivation
- Impulsivity
- Irritability
- Agitation
- Aggression
- Errors of judgement
- Decreased abstract thinking
- Attention and concentration
- Difficulties in planning and problem-solving
- Memory issues
- Impaired activities of daily living

Brief Mental State Examination
- How has your mood been?
- How is your sleep?
- How is your appetite?
- Anhedonia
- Do you see things when there is no one around you?
- Do you hear voices when there is no one around you?

Risk
- Any suicidal thoughts?
- Any thoughts of harming anyone else?
- Do you take alcohol in excess?
- Do you take recreational drugs?

- Have you seen a psychiatrist previously [8]?

References

1. World Health Organization. Dissociative disorders (BlockL1-6B6). 6B60.6 Dissociative neurological symptom disorder, with paresis or weakness. ICD-11 International Classification of Diseases—mortality and morbidity statistics. 11th revision ed. World Health Organization; 2018. p. 52.
2. Semple D, Smyth R. Chapter 2. Psychiatric assessment. History. Mental state examination. Oxford handbook of psychiatry. 3rd ed. Oxford University Press; 2017. p. 42–44.
3. World Health Organization. Anxiety or fear-related disorders (BlockL1-6B0). 6B21 Body dysmorphic disorder. ICD-11 International Classification of Diseases—mortality and morbidity statistics. 11th revision ed. World Health Organization; 2018. p. 44.
4. World Health Organization. Anxiety or fear-related disorders (BlockL1-6B0). 6B23 Hypochondriasis. ICD-11 International Classification of Diseases—mortality and morbidity statistics. 11th revision ed. World Health Organization; 2018. p. 45.
5. World Health Organization. Disorders of bodily distress or bodily experience (BlockL1-6C2). 6C20 Bodily distress disorder. ICD-11 International Classification of Diseases—mortality and morbidity statistics. 11th revision ed. World Health Organization; 2018. p. 63.
6. Semple D, Smyth R. Liaison psychiatry. Parasuicide assessment. Oxford handbook of psychiatry. 3rd ed. Oxford University Press; 2017. p. 784.
7. Taylor DM, Barnes T, Young A. Catatonia. The Maudsley prescribing guidelines in psychiatry. 14th ed. Wiley Blackwell; 2021. p. 135.
8. National Institute for Health and Care Excellence. Head injury: assessment and early management clinical guideline [CG176]. 2019. https://www.nice.org.uk/guidance/cg176/chapter/Recommendations#pre-hospital-assessment-advice-and-referral-to-hospital. Accessed September.

Eating Disorders

Bulimia Nervosa

Scenario

22-year-old Georgina Irvine has been referred by the GP since she has been having some issues with eating.

Task

Take a relevant history, and assess prognostic factors for her condition.

Approach

Hello, I am Dr. _____. I am a psychiatrist. I understand you have been referred by the GP with a few issues around your eating habits. Please could you tell me more?

History of Presenting Complaint
- What is your height?
- May I ask how much you weigh?
- Do you know what your body mass index is?
- Do you feel you are overweight?
- What is your ideal weight?
- Are there certain parts of your body that you are particularly unhappy with?
- May I ask if you have issues with your body image?

All names and scenarios mentioned in this book are fictitious. Any resemblance to actual individuals or backgrounds is entirely conincidental.

© The Author(s), under exclusive license to Springer Nature Switzerland AG 2023

N. Sivaswamy, *Prepare for the MRCPsych CASC Exam*, https://doi.org/10.1007/978-3-031-31019-5_6

Elicit the Details of Eating Disorder
- Describe your eating pattern in a typical day.
- Do you avoid particular foods and why?
- Do you restrict fluids and why?
- Do you binge eat: by that I mean do you eat a large amount of food in a short span of time?
- Describe what you might eat in a typical binge?
- How long does the episode of binging last?
- How often do you binge?
- How do you feel before you binge?
- How do you feel after you binge?
- Are you able to identify a particular trigger for the binge eating?
- Have you ever tried to make yourself sick?
- How do you do this?
- How often do you do this?
- Why do you do this?
- Do you use laxatives, purgatives, emetics and appetite suppressants to aid weight loss?
- Do you fast for a day or more?
- Do you exercise—how many hours a day and how often?
- Have you noticed any weakness, constipation, tiredness and dizziness [1]?

Prognostic Factors
- Are you menstruating regularly?
- Has there been a time where you have not had your periods?
- What was the longest time that you have not had your periods?
- Any stressors at home or work?
- Any relationship difficulties?
- How is your relationship with your parents?
- How would you describe your personality—would you say you were a perfectionist?
- How would you describe your self-esteem?
- When did you first start to have issues around your eating habits?
- How long after developing issues around your eating did you see a doctor?
- Have you been given a diagnosis of eating disorder [2]?

Impact and Coping
This sounds really difficult for you. How has this impacted on your

- Relationships
- Work

  With all this going on, how have you been coping?

- May I ask if you take alcohol in excess?
- May I ask if you take any recreational drugs at all?

Psychiatric History

Have you seen a psychiatrist in the past?

Medical History

Do you have any physical health issues?

Family History

Anyone in the family with a diagnosis of eating disorders?

Medication and Compliance

Do you take any regular medication?

Brief Mental State Examination

Ask about mood, sleep, anhedonia, generalised anxiety, and auditory and visual hallucinations.

Risk Assessment

Suicidal thoughts or plans, thoughts of harming others and deliberate self-harm [3]

Station-Specific Points

- This is a long station with different areas to explore, so make judicious use of time.

Anorexia Nervosa

Scenario

19-year-old Edwina Adams has been an inpatient in the eating disorder unit for the past 3 months following a diagnosis of anorexia nervosa. She has made a good recovery and will be discharged shortly. You have just started your placement in the unit and have been asked to speak to her by the consultant.

Task

Assess the prognostic factors for her condition.

Approach

Hello, I am Dr. ____. I am a psychiatrist. May I ask you a few questions please?

Prognostic Factors
- What is your current weight?
- What was your weight at the time of admission?
- What age were you when you first developed anorexia?
- When did you first start to have issues around your eating habits?
- How long after developing issues around your eating were you given a diagnosis?
- Have you always had eating issues or have you had periods of normal eating?
- Have you ever had any binge eating behaviours?
- Have you had any purging behaviours?
- Are you menstruating regularly?
- Has there been a time where you have not had your periods?
- What was the longest time that you have not had your periods?
- Have you ever experienced any physical health problems like weakness, constipation, dizziness and lethargy?
- Any stressors at home or work?
- Any relationship difficulties?
- How would you describe your personality—would you say you were a perfectionist?
- How is your relationship with your parents?
- What do they do for a living?
- Were you working or studying prior to admission?
- Have you felt your parents have high expectations of you?
- Have you felt they are overinvolved in your life?
- Have you ever had difficulty communicating your needs and felt you deprived yourself of food as a means of communication [4]?

Substance and Alcohol Misuse
- May I ask if you take alcohol in excess?
- May I ask if you take any recreational drugs?

Psychiatric History
Have you seen a psychiatrist in the past?

Medical History
Do you have any physical health issues?

Medication and Compliance
Do you take any regular medication?

Family History
Anyone in the family with a diagnosis of eating disorders?

Brief Mental State Examination
Ask about mood, sleep, anhedonia, generalised anxiety, and auditory and visual hallucinations.

Risk Assessment

Suicidal thoughts or plans, thoughts of harming others and deliberate self-harm [3]

Station-Specific Points

The family dynamics should be explored sensitively.

Refeeding Syndrome

Scenario

Luke Nisbet is a community psychiatric nurse working with the eating disorder team. He wants to discuss 17-year-old Alice Parish with you as he is concerned about her following a review appointment today.

Task

Speak to the nurse, and address his concerns.
   Explain the diagnosis, and formulate a management plan.

Approach

Hello, I am Dr. ____. I am a psychiatrist. I understand you have some concerns about Alice. Please could you tell me more?
- Speak to Luke, and elicit all relevant information including his concerns about Alice.

Explain the Diagnosis
- From our discussion, it appears that she has developed a condition called refeeding syndrome.
- It is a disorder of fluid and salt balance in the body. The body depends on glucose obtained from carbohydrates for energy.
- When the body is starved of nutrition, it runs out of carbohydrates and then starts breaking down fats and protein to provide energy.
- This process results in the shift of salts including potassium and phosphate from within the cell into the bloodstream.
- On refeeding, when the body suddenly receives a lot of food, the salts move from the bloodstream back into the cells, which results in a deficit of these salts in the bloodstream.
- The heart is unable to cope with the increased load, and there is an increased risk of heart failure with problems like oedema.
- The low levels of potassium can cause disturbances in heart rhythm.
- The low phosphate levels can cause muscular problems.

Management

1. This is a medical emergency that can be life-threatening.
2. The patient should be immediately asked to report to the nearest A&E.
3. Refeeding syndrome cannot be managed as an outpatient, and she has to be treated in a medical hospital.
4. Perform all relevant blood investigations and an ECG.
5. Frequent check of electrolytes with correction of electrolyte imbalance.
6. Prescribe thiamine and vitamin B complex.
7. A dietician should be involved.
8. Aim for weight gain of no more than 0.5 kg to 1 kg per week.
9. Multidisciplinary team approach involving gastroenterologist, dietician and psychiatrist.
10. Psychoeducation to family [5].

Station-Specific Points

- Jargon can be used while speaking to a medical colleague.
- Emphasise that this is a medical emergency and the individual has to report to hospital immediately.

Anorexia Nervosa and Mental Health Act

Scenario

19-year-old Marina Lambeth has been admitted to the hospital after she lost consciousness, and her flatmate reported that she has not been eating or drinking for the last 4 days. She has been diagnosed with anorexia nervosa. Her mother is waiting to speak to you. Marina has consented for information to be shared with her mother.

Task

Speak to her mother Mrs. Lambeth and answer her questions.

Approach

Hello, I am Dr. ____. I am a psychiatrist. I understand you are here to speak to me about your daughter.

- Please may I clarify what you know so far?
- She appears to have a diagnosis of anorexia nervosa, which is a type of eating disorder. Have you heard of this before?

- It is a type of eating disorder where a person has an intense fear of gaining weight. They use various methods like dieting, overexercising, counting calories, excluding certain foods and using medications that make them vomit or cause loose stools.
- The lack of nutrition can cause physical problems like fatigue, hair loss, softening of the bones, irregular periods and changes in the salts in their body.
- Feeding against the will of the patient is an intervention of last resort.
- The Mental Health Act can only be used when the severe lack of nutrition has affected their ability to make decisions and there is a risk to their life.
- The Mental Health Act can only be used following a detailed assessment of mental state.
- No one else can give consent on behalf of the individual who is requiring treatment.

Management
1. Individuals can be managed in the community with intense physical health monitoring, dietician input and regular follow-up with the eating disorder service.
2. Admission in hospital can be considered if there is rapid weight loss with salt imbalances and physical health problems.
3. Dietician input is vital to devising a meal plan with a goal of gradual weight restoration.
4. Family-based therapeutic interventions.
5. Psychoeducation and support to family/carers [5].

References

1. World Health Organization. Feeding or eating disorders (BlockL1-6B8). 6B81 Bulimia nervosa. ICD-11 International Classification of Diseases—mortality and morbidity statistics. 11th revision ed. World Health Organization; 2018. p. 59.
2. Steinhausen HC, Weber S. The outcome of Bulimia nervosa: findings from one-quarter century of research. Am J Psychiatry. 2009;166(12):1331.
3. Semple D, Smyth R. Chapter 2. Psychiatric assessment. History. Mental state examination. Oxford handbook of psychiatry. 3rd ed. Oxford University Press; 2017. p. 42–44.
4. Papadopoulos F, Ekbom A, Brandt L, Ekselius L. Excess mortality, causes of death and prognostic factors in anorexia nervosa. Br J Psychiatry. 2018;194(1):10.
5. Royal College of Psychiatrists London. Medical emergencies in eating disorders: guidance on recognition and management. College Report. 2022;CR233.

Paedophilia

Scenario

37-year-old Gary Moore has been brought by the police for psychiatric assessment after his neighbour 9-year-old Debra Hastings accused him of touching her inappropriately.

Task

Take a relevant history, and perform a risk assessment.

Approach

Hello, I am Dr. _____. I am a psychiatrist. I understand you have been brought in by the police after your neighbour made some allegations. I am going to ask you a few questions, some of which may be of a personal nature.

History of Index Incident
- Please could you tell me the circumstances that brought you to the attention of the police?
- Has anything similar happened in the past? Elicit details.
- I understand Debra is your neighbour—how well do you know her?
- How often does she visit your house?

© The Author(s), under exclusive license to Springer Nature Switzerland AG 2023

N. Sivaswamy, *Prepare for the MRCPsych CASC Exam*, https://doi.org/10.1007/978-3-031-31019-5_7

- Is it with her parents' knowledge that she visits you?
- When she spent time at your house, did you touch her inappropriately?
- Did you masturbate when she was in your house?
- Were you sexually aroused when she was visiting your house?
- What is your explanation for what happened?
- Do you think what you did was wrong?
- Do you feel guilty for what happened?
- Have you thought about the consequences of your behaviour?
- What are your thoughts on Debra's feelings [1]?

Psychosexual History
- Are you in a relationship at present?
- Any issues in your current relationship/previous relationships?
- Do you masturbate?
- Do you have any sexual fantasies?
- Do you have any unconventional sexual practices?
- Are you sexually attracted to children?
- Do you use pornography?
- Do you use child pornography?

Psychiatric History
Have you seen a psychiatrist in the past?

Medical History
Do you have any medical problems?

Medication and Compliance
Do you take any regular medication?

Forensic History
- Any problems with the police?
- Any charges?
- Any convictions?
- Any charges for sexual offences?
- Any charges as a juvenile?

Substance and Alcohol Misuse
- Do you take any recreational drugs?
- Do you take alcohol in excess?

Brief Mental State Examination
Ask about mood, sleep, appetite, anhedonia, generalised anxiety, auditory and visual hallucinations and insight.

Risk Assessment

- Suicidal thoughts or plans
- Deliberate self-harm
- Thoughts of harming others—especially the person who complained against him
- What is your line of work—do you come into contact with children as part of your work?
- Are there any other children that you meet regularly?
- Does Debra have any siblings that also visit you?
- Have you ever tried to meet Debra without her parents' knowledge?
- Was it your intent to groom Debra or any other children?

Social History

- Do you have any friends or family who can offer you support?
- How was your childhood—any difficult incidents of abuse or neglect?
- How would you describe your personality?
- Do you have any stressors in your life [2]?

Station-Specific Points

- Perform a risk assessment, especially contact with other children.
- Elicit a forensic history and psychosexual history.

Exhibitionism

Scenario

82-year-old Nathan Black was brought by the police following a complaint that he exposed himself to a group of children in the local park.

Task

Take a relevant history.

Approach

Hello, I am Dr. _____. I am a psychiatrist. I understand you have been brought in by the police. I am going to ask you a few questions, some of which may be of a personal nature.

History of Index Incident
- Please could you tell me the circumstances that brought you to the attention of the police?
- Elicit details of the incident.
- Has anything similar happened in the past?
- What is your explanation for what happened?
- Do you think what you did was wrong?
- Do you feel guilty for what happened?
- Have you thought about the consequences of your behaviour?
- What are your thoughts on the feelings of those children?
- What was your intent—was it to get sexually aroused yourself or was it to get the children aroused?
- At the time did you masturbate?
- At the time was your penis erect or flaccid [3]?

Psychosexual History
- Are you in a relationship at present?
- Any issues in your current relationship/previous relationships?
- Do you masturbate?
- Do you have any sexual fantasies?
- Do you have any unconventional sexual practices?
- Are you sexually attracted to children?
- Do you use pornography?
- Do you use child pornography?

Psychiatric History
Have you seen a psychiatrist in the past?

Medical History
Do you have any medical problems?

Medication and Compliance
Do you take any regular medication?

Forensic History
- Any problems with the police?
- Any charges?
- Any convictions?
- Any charges for sexual offences?
- Any charges as a juvenile?

Substance and Alcohol Misuse
- Do you take any recreational drugs?
- Do you take alcohol in excess?

Brief Mental State Examination

Ask about mood, sleep, appetite, anhedonia, generalised anxiety, auditory and visual hallucinations and insight.

Ask about memory and concentration.

Risk Assessment

- Suicidal thoughts or plans
- Deliberate self-harm
- Thoughts of harming others—especially the person who complained against him
- What is your line of work?
- Do you come into contact with children as part of your work?
- Do you have any other children that you meet regularly?

Social History

- Do you have any friends or family who can offer you support?
- How was your childhood—any difficult incidents of abuse or neglect?
- How would you describe your personality?
- Do you have any stressors in your life [2]?

Station-Specific Points

- Anticipate that the actor may be embarrassed by his behaviour.
- Perform a risk assessment.
- Elicit a forensic history and psychosexual history.

Indecent Exposure

Scenario

61-year-old Winston Gates was brought by the police following a complaint by his neighbour 49-year-old Jessica Parks that he exposed himself to her while she was in her garden.

Task

Take a relevant history.

Approach

Hello, I am Dr. _____. I am a psychiatrist. I understand you have been brought in by the police. I am going to ask you a few questions, some of which may be of a personal nature.

History of Index Incident
- Please could you tell me the circumstances that brought you to the attention of the police?
- Elicit details of the incident.
- Has anything similar happened in the past?
- What is your explanation for what happened?
- Do you think what you did was wrong?
- Do you feel guilty for what happened?
- Have you thought about the consequences of your behaviour?
- What are your thoughts on the feelings of your neighbour?
- What was your intent—was it to get aroused or was it to get your neighbour aroused?
- At the time did you masturbate?
- At the time was your penis erect or flaccid [4]?

Psychosexual History
- Are you in a relationship at present?
- Any issues in your current relationship/previous relationships?
- Do you masturbate?
- Do you have any sexual fantasies?
- Do you have any unconventional sexual practices?
- Are you sexually attracted to children?
- Do you use pornography?
- Do you use child pornography?

Psychiatric History

Have you seen a psychiatrist in the past?

Medical History

Do you have any medical problems?

Medication and Compliance

Do you take any regular medication?

Forensic History

Any problems with the police?

- Any charges?
- Any convictions?
- Any charges for sexual offences?
- Any charges as a juvenile?

Substance and Alcohol Misuse

- Do you take any recreational drugs?
- Do you take alcohol in excess?

Brief Mental State Examination

Ask about mood, sleep, appetite, anhedonia, generalised anxiety, auditory and visual hallucinations, insight, memory and concentration.

Risk Assessment

- Suicidal thoughts or plans
- Deliberate self-harm
- Thoughts of harming others—especially the person who complained against him

Social History

- Do you have any friends or family who can offer you support?
- How was your childhood—any difficult incidents of abuse or neglect?
- How would you describe your personality?
- What is your occupation [2]?

Station-Specific Points

- Anticipate that the actor may not be forthcoming with information.
- Elicit a forensic history and psychosexual history.

Morbid Jealousy

Scenario

33-year-old John Hodges was referred by the GP after he expressed increasing anger due to his belief that his partner Jane is having an affair. The GP has discussed with Jane who vehemently denies infidelity on her part.

Task

Take a relevant history.

Approach

Hello, I am Dr. _____. I am a psychiatrist. I understand you have been referred by the GP as you voiced concerns about your partner's infidelity. I am sorry to hear that. Please could you tell me more?

History of Presenting Complaint

- Explore the circumstances leading to his current presentation.
- Elicit details of his concerns.

- When did you start thinking this way?
- What was happening in your life at that time?
- Has anything similar happened in the past?
- Why do you suspect your partner is having an affair?
- Who do you think she is having an affair with?
- How do you know this is true?
- Have you seen them together?

Intense Seeking Behaviours to Find Evidence of Her Infidelity

- Have you followed your partner?
- Have you followed the person you think she is having an affair with?
- Have you searched her handbag or mobile phone?

Impact

How has feeling this way impacted on your work and life?

Psychiatric History

Have you seen a psychiatrist in the past?

Family History

Anyone in the family with any mental or physical health issues?

Medical History

Do you have any medical problems?

Medication and Compliance

Do you take any regular medication?

Forensic History

- Any problems with the police?
- Any charges?
- Any convictions?
- Any charges for domestic violence?

Substance and Alcohol Misuse

- Do you take any recreational drugs?
- Do you take alcohol in excess?

Brief Mental State Examination

- Ask about mood, sleep, appetite, anhedonia, generalised anxiety, auditory and visual hallucinations and insight.
- Did you start thinking this way out of the blue or following an unusual experience?
- How convinced are you that your partner is having an affair?
- Could there be any other explanation?
- Have you discussed this with anyone? What did they say?

Risk Assessment
- Do you have any thoughts of ending your life?
- Have you had any thoughts of harming your partner?
- Have you had any thoughts of harming the person you believe your partner is having an affair with?
- Has domestic violence been an issue in your relationship?
- Have you ever made any threats of violence?
- Do you have access to any weapons?
- Are there any children at home?

Social History
- May I ask if you have any marital problems?
- May I ask if you have any sexual problems?
- How was your childhood—any difficult incidents of abuse or neglect?
- How would you describe your personality [5]?

Erotomania

Scenario

41-year-old Steven Pulman has come to the reception of the local hospital demanding to speak to Maya Myers, a staff nurse in the psychiatric ward. The reception staff have asked you as the psychiatrist on call to speak to him due to his demands to see Maya.

Task

Take a relevant history, and perform a risk assessment.

Approach

Hello, I am Dr. _____. I am a psychiatrist. I understand you are here to see Maya, one of the staff nurses in the hospital. May I ask why you would like to see her?

History of Presenting Complaint
- May I ask how you met her?
- Was it through your mental health needs?
- Are you in love with her?
- Do you think she is in love with you?
- How do you know she is in love with you?
- Has she told you this?
- Do you have any evidence to support these thoughts?

- Is this the first time you have tried to make contact with her?
- Do you know her home address, mobile number or email address?
- Have you been observing her or following her?
- May I ask if you have had any sexual fantasies about her?
- Have you had similar thoughts about anyone else previously? Elicit details.
- Do you know if she has a partner already?
- If she does have a partner, how will you handle this?
- How convinced are you that she reciprocates your feelings?
- Could she have been doing her job and you misinterpreted this?
- Do you think there is an alternate explanation for you thinking this way?

Impact and Coping
How has feeling this impacted your work and life?

Psychiatric History
Have you seen a psychiatrist in the past?

Medical History
Do you have any medical problems?

Medication and Compliance
Do you take any regular medication?

Forensic History
- Any problems with the police?
- Any charges?
- Any convictions?

Substance and Alcohol Misuse
- Do you take any recreational drugs?
- Do you take alcohol in excess?

Brief Mental State Examination
Ask about mood, sleep, appetite, anhedonia, generalised anxiety, auditory and visual hallucinations and insight.

Risk Assessment
- What do you intend to do if you meet her?
- What would you do if your feelings were not reciprocated?
- Is there a chance you might harm her in any way?
- Is there a chance you might harm her partner if she had one?
- Is there a chance you might harm yourself?
- Do you have thoughts of violence or suicide?
- Do you have any thoughts of harming anyone else?
- Do you have access to any weapons?

- What would you do if you cannot see her now?
- What would you do if she says she does not want to see you?

Social History

I am going to ask you a few personal questions.

- May I ask if you have any sexual problems?
- How was your childhood—any difficult incidents of abuse or neglect?
- How would you describe your personality [6]?

Station-Specific Points

- The actor will frequently ask to see the staff nurse—manage this tactfully to continue the assessment.
- Elicit a forensic history, and perform a risk assessment.

Future Violence Risk Assessment

Scenario

47-year-old Donald Wick has been brought in by the police to the psychiatric hospital after he assaulted a man in the pub. The police have requested a violence risk assessment.

Task

Perform a future violence risk assessment.

Approach

Hello, I am Dr. _____. I am a psychiatrist.

- Can you tell me a little more about the circumstances that brought you to the attention of the police?
- What was your intent when you did this?
- What are your views about what happened—do you feel anger, remorse or guilt?
- Has anything like this happened before?
- Do you have any thoughts of harming yourself?
- Any suicidal thoughts?
- Do you have any thoughts of harming anyone else?
- May I check if there are any children living with you or who visit you?

- Do you have any particular people that you have thoughts of hurting?
- How do you plan to do this?
- When do you plan to do this?
- Where will you do this?
- How long have you been thinking this way?
- Do you have access to any weapons?

Psychiatric History

- Have you seen a psychiatrist before?
- Have you been admitted to a psychiatric hospital before?

Medical History

- Do you have any medical problems?
- Do you take medication as prescribed?

Substance and Alcohol Misuse

- Do you take alcohol in excess?
- Do you use any recreational drugs?

Forensic History

- Do you have any trouble with the police?
- Any convictions?
- Any charges?
- Have there been any particular victims?
- Describe your personality—impulsive/short tempered.
- Any relationship issues?

Brief Mental State Examination

- Ask about mood, sleep, appetite and anhedonia.
- Do you hear voices when there is no one around?
- Do you see things when there is no one around?
- Thought disorder?
- Delusional beliefs [7]?

Fire Setting

Scenario

35-year-old Helen Wallace resides in sheltered accommodation. She set a fire in her room due to which the fire service was called and the entire accommodation evacuated. Police were asked to attend and requested a psychiatric review as there have been similar instances previously.

Task

Explore possible reasons for her fire-setting behaviours, and perform a risk assessment.

Approach

Hello, I am Dr. ___. I am a psychiatrist. I understand you set a fire in your accommodation. I would like to ask you a few questions about this please.

- What were you doing before you set the fire?
- What did you do exactly?
- Were you hurt at all?
- Do you know if anyone else was hurt?
- Was it planned or impulsive?
- What was your intent?
- Did you take any precautions to prevent anyone finding out that you are setting a fire?
- How did you feel after lighting the fire?
- Did you feel any pleasure?
- Were you sexually aroused?
- Do you take responsibility for what you did?
- Do you feel guilty or remorseful for setting the fire?
- What did you do after you started the fire?
- Why did you set the fire—curiosity, experimentation or cry for help?
- When did the fire-setting behaviour first start?
- What was happening in your life at that time?

Risk Assessment
- Do you still have thoughts of starting a fire at present?
- Any future plans to set fire to things?
- Any suicidal thoughts?
- Any thoughts of harming anyone else?

Brief Mental State Examination
Enquire about mood, sleep, appetite, anhedonia, generalised anxiety and seeing things/hearing voices.

Psychiatric History
Have you seen a psychiatrist before?

Substance and Alcohol Misuse
- Do you take alcohol in excess?
- Any recreational drug use at all?

Forensic History
Have you had any trouble with the police before?

Childhood
When you think about your childhood, is there anything that stands out for you?

Social History
Friends/family support [8]

Stalking

Scenario

47-year-old Alfred Banks has been brought by the police for psychiatric assessment after he was found breaking and entering a property.

Task

Take a relevant history, and perform a risk assessment.

Approach

Hello, I am Dr. _____. I am a psychiatrist. I understand you have been brought in by the police.

History of Index Incident
- Please could you tell me the circumstances that brought you to the attention of the police?
- Has anything similar happened in the past?
- Whom does the property you broke into belong to?
- How do you know this person?
- What is your explanation for breaking into the house?
- What was your intent?
- Do you think what you did was wrong?
- Do you feel guilty for what happened?
- Have you thought about the consequences of your behaviour?
- What are your thoughts on that person's feelings?

Psychiatric History
Have you seen a psychiatrist in the past?

Family History
Anyone in the family with any mental or physical health issues?

Medical History
Do you have any medical problems?

Medication and Compliance
Do you take any regular medication?

Forensic History
- Any problems with the police?
- Any charges?
- Any convictions?

Substance and Alcohol Misuse
- Do you take any recreational drugs?
- Do you take alcohol in excess?

Brief Mental State Examination
- Ask about mood, sleep, appetite, anhedonia, generalised anxiety, auditory and visual hallucinations and passivity.
- Elicit details of any delusions.
- Elicit conviction and fixity of beliefs.

Risk Assessment
- Suicidal thoughts or plans
- Deliberate self-harm
- Thoughts of harming others—especially the person who resides in the property
- Access to weapons

Social History
Do you have any friends or family who can offer you support?
How was your childhood—any difficult incidents of abuse or neglect?
How would you describe your personality?
Do you have any stressors in your life [6]?

Station-Specific Points

Perform a mental state examination and risk assessment.

Drug-Induced Psychosis

Scenario

33-year-old David Harrison is in prison serving a sentence for drug possession. He was moved to the hospital wing of the prison 1 day ago due to agitation and paranoid behaviour. The hospital staff have requested a psychiatric review.

Task

Take a brief history, and discuss the management options with Percy who is the staff nurse in the hospital wing of the prison.

Approach

Hello, I am Dr. _____. I am a psychiatrist. I understand Mr. Harrison is currently in the hospital wing of the prison.

Brief History
- How was his presentation before he was brought to the hospital wing?
- How is this different from his usual presentation?
- Does he have a psychiatric diagnosis?
- Any medical problems?
- Is he on any medication and how is the compliance?
- Is there a possibility he might have used recreational drugs while in prison?
- Mental state examination: Did he appear depressed, or did he appear to be hearing things or seeing things that are not really there? Enquire about thought disorder and delusional beliefs. Has he voiced thoughts of harming himself or anyone else?

Management
1. Mr. Harrison has to remain in the hospital wing of the prison as he requires a period of observation.
2. Risks: possible risk to others if he is paranoid about being harmed by others. Passivity symptoms are of particular concern. He is also at risk of retribution from others if he were to act on his paranoid thoughts.
3. I will meet him and perform an assessment of mental state.
4. Perform a urine drug screen.
5. Obtain collateral history from GP and other staff here who know him well.
6. Medication can be considered if appropriate after all the above [9].

References

1. World Health Organization. Paraphilic disorders (BlockL1-6D3). 6D32 Pedophilic disorder. ICD-11 International Classification of Diseases—mortality and morbidity statistics. 11th revision ed. World Health Organization; 2018. p. 178.
2. Russell K, Darjee R. Practical assessment and management of risk in sexual offenders. Adv Psychiatr Treat. 2013;19(1):56.
3. World Health Organization. Paraphilic disorders (BlockL1-6D3). 6D30 Exhibitionistic disorder. ICD-11 International Classification of Diseases—mortality and morbidity statistics. 11th revision ed. World Health Organization; 2018. p. 177.
4. Darjee R, Russell K. What clinicians need to know before assessing risk in sexual offenders. Adv Psychiatr Treat. 2012;18(6):467.
5. Kingham M, Gordon H. Aspects of morbid jealousy. Adv Psychiatr Treat. 2004;10(3):207.
6. Mullen PE, Pathé M, Purcell R. The management of stalkers. Adv Psychiatr Treat. 2001;7(5):335.
7. Semple D, Smyth R. Forensic psychiatry. Assessing risk of violence. Oxford handbook of psychiatry. 3rd ed. Oxford University Press; 2017. p. 692.
8. Burton P, McNiel D, Binder R. Firesetting, arson, pyromania, and the forensic mental health expert. J Am Acad Psychiatry Law. 2012;40(3):355.
9. Semple D, Smyth R. Severe behavioural disturbance. Oxford handbook of psychiatry. 3rd ed. Oxford University Press; 2017. p. 988.

Psychotherapy

Systematic Desensitisation

Scenario

42-year-old Shauna Forsythe has been diagnosed with agoraphobia by the GP and has been referred to psychiatric services to discuss the psychological therapy for her condition.

Task

Explain the psychological therapy for her condition.

Approach

Hello, I am Dr. _____. I am a psychiatrist. I understand you have been diagnosed with agoraphobia and have been referred by the GP to discuss talking therapy.

Explain the Psychological Therapy
- The psychological therapy is called systematic desensitisation.
- It is a simple and highly effective technique.
- It is based on cognitive behavioural therapy looking at the thought behaviour mood link.
- Evidence shows that most individuals respond positively to this form of therapy; however, active participation of the individual is required.

All names and scenarios mentioned in this book are fictitious. Any resemblance to actual individuals or backgrounds is entirely conincidental.

© The Author(s), under exclusive license to Springer Nature Switzerland AG 2023

N. Sivaswamy, *Prepare for the MRCPsych CASC Exam*, https://doi.org/10.1007/978-3-031-31019-5_8

- The goals of therapy belong to the individual.
- A qualified therapist works with the client to develop an individualised plan involving a graded program of exposure to tasks in incremental steps. This involves making a list of tasks from the least to the most anxiety-provoking circumstances. You may think of this as a ladder.
- The therapist will teach you deep breathing and muscle relaxation techniques, and you will be encouraged to use these techniques prior to each step on the list.
- You will start on the lowest rung of the ladder and slowly move your way up each step while using the deep breathing and muscle relaxation techniques.
- If you have difficulty in any step, you will move one step down the ladder, and once you are comfortable you will slowly move up the list again.
- For example, you will initially be encouraged to come out of your room, then come downstairs, then to the front door, walk to the gate and so on.
- The therapy is 8–12 regular weekly sessions with each session lasting about an hour. The exact number of sessions can be agreed with the therapist.
- If you have difficulty attending the clinic for the initial sessions, the therapist can visit your home.
- The sessions are strictly time limited.
- Last few sessions will focus on relapse prevention, that is, if you were starting to feel unwell again, how you would manage this confidently.
- You will be given homework tasks, and your family can help you complete these tasks [1].
- May I ask how motivated you are to engage in this therapy?
- Family support is important.
- Psychoeducation.
- Offer leaflets.

Station-Specific Points

Chunk and check.

Exposure Response Prevention

Scenario

34-year-old Sally Dupont has been diagnosed with obsessive compulsive disorder (OCD) and has been referred to you to discuss psychological therapy for her condition.

Task

Explain the psychological therapy for her condition.

Approach

Hello, I am Dr. ____. I am a psychiatrist. I understand you have been diagnosed with OCD and have been referred by the GP to discuss talking therapy.

Explain the Psychological Therapy
- The psychological therapy is called exposure response prevention.
- It is a simple and highly effective technique.
- It is based on cognitive behavioural therapy looking at the thought behaviour mood link.
- Evidence shows that most individuals respond positively to this form of therapy; however, active participation of the individual is required.
- The goals of therapy belong to the individual.
- A qualified therapist works with the client to develop an individualised plan involving a graded programme of exposure to tasks. This includes setting specific targets.
- The therapist will teach you deep breathing and muscle relaxation techniques, and you will be encouraged to use these techniques to manage the anxiety.
- The idea is that you will slowly learn to manage and resist the unhelpful thoughts in your mind.
- The associated anxiety will reduce over time with repeated attempts.
- You can practise by imagining the situation in your mind; however, it is more effective if done in reality.
- The therapy is 8–12 regular weekly sessions with each session lasting about an hour. The exact number of sessions can be agreed with the therapist based on clinical requirement [2].
- May I ask how motivated you are to engage in this therapy?
- Family support is important.
- Psychoeducation.
- Offer leaflets.

Station-Specific Points

- Chunk and check.
- The role player may become anxious, and it is important to be reassuring and contain their anxiety while managing your time well.

Displacement Reaction

Scenario

37-year-old Theodore McCarthy has been having some issues at work and has been referred by his GP who is of the opinion that there may be a psychological aspect to his presentation.

Task

Take a history to identify the defence mechanism.

Approach

Hello, I am Dr. _____. I am a psychiatrist. I understand you have been having some difficulties. I am sorry to hear that. Please could you tell me more?

History of Presenting Complaint
- When did all this first start?
- What was happening in your life at that time?
- Has anything like this happened before?
- Are there any triggers that make you think this way?
- Is there anything that makes these thoughts better or worse?
- May I ask about your personal life—are you in a relationship?
- Do you have any issues or worries about your relationship with your partner?
- Have you discussed this with your partner?

Impact and Coping
This sounds really difficult for you. How has this impacted on your

- Relationship
- Work

    With all this going on, how have you been coping?

- May I ask if you take alcohol in excess?
- May I ask if you take any recreational drugs?

Psychiatric History
Have you seen a psychiatrist in the past?

Family History
Anyone in the family with any mental or physical health issues?

Medication and Compliance
Do you take any regular medication?
    Do you take the medication as prescribed?

Brief Mental State Examination
Ask about mood, sleep, appetite, anhedonia, generalised anxiety, and auditory and visual hallucinations.

Risk Assessment
- Suicidal thoughts
- Deliberate self-harm
- Thoughts of harming your partner
- Thoughts of harming the person your partner is having an affair with [3]

Explain the Psychological Phenomena
It appears you have a condition called displacement reaction. You are having some issues in your personal life that you feel unable to discuss with your partner and therefore you are displacing these emotions onto your work [4].

Station-Specific Points

- The role player will not be forthcoming with information.
- Remember to sensitively explore the difficulties in his life.
- Explain the diagnosis in simple language.

Transference Reaction

Scenario

26-year-old Mary Aitken would like to discontinue her psychotherapy sessions. You have been asked to speak to her as the psychiatrist on call.

Task

Speak to her, and identify the psychological issue.

Approach

Hello, I am Dr. _____. I am a psychiatrist. I understand you want to discontinue your therapy sessions. I am sorry to hear that. Please could you tell me more?

History of Presenting Complaint
- What form of therapy are you engaged in?
- Why have you been started on this therapy?
- Do you have a psychiatric diagnosis?
- Are you on any medication and do you take it as prescribed?
- May I ask if you take alcohol excess?
- May I ask if you take any recreational drugs?

Patient Factors
- Do you have any difficulty attending the session due to the date/time being unsuitable?
- Do you have issues getting time off work to attend sessions?
- Are there childcare issues that conflict with your attending sessions?
- Any transportation issues?

Therapist Factors
- Do you think the therapist is a competent professional?
- Do you know if the therapist is moving away or perhaps moving jobs?
- Have there been frequent cancellation of sessions that have been inconvenient?

When we engage in psychological therapy, we share a lot of personal information with the therapist which can cause various emotions to surface and we can be reminded of people from the past. Usually, the person will be an important figure in our lives like a parent.

Have your therapy sessions reminded you of a figure from your past?

Explain the Psychological Phenomena
- It appears you have a condition called transference reaction, whereby emotions from the past related to an important figure in your life are being mirrored or transferred on to present relationships, namely the therapist.

The decision about continuing or ending therapy is yours to make; however, I would suggest discussing this with your therapist before you decide [5].

Station-Specific Points

Chunk and check.

Interpersonal Therapy

Scenario

45-year-old June Carter has been diagnosed with depression and started on fluoxetine by the GP. She has been referred to the psychotherapy service to assess suitability for interpersonal therapy.

Task

Assess suitability for interpersonal therapy.

Approach

Hello, I am Dr. _____. I am a psychiatrist. I understand you have been diagnosed with depression by your GP and started on medication, and we are here today to assess if you are suitable for interpersonal therapy.

Assess for Core Symptoms of Depression

Ask about

- Mood
- Sleep
- Appetite
- Anhedonia
- Memory
- Concentration
- Suicidal thoughts

Assess for Selection Criteria

- Mild-to-moderate depression
- May I check you are not admitted in any hospital and have come to see me as an outpatient?
- Non-psychotic depressive illness: Have you ever had any unusual experiences like hearing voices or seeing things when there is no one around you?
- Non-bipolar depressive illness: Have you ever felt exceedingly happy?

Identify Interpersonal Problem Areas

- May I ask who are the members of your family?
- How is your relationship with your husband/partner?
- Do you have any children and are they presently at home?
- How is your relationship with your children?
- Do you have any close friends and how has your relationship with them been?
- Have you had any recent disputes or conflicts with anyone close to you?
- Do you take any recreational drugs or alcohol?

Recent Changes

- Children moving away
- Graduation
- Separation or divorce
- Any other stressful events
- Physical health issues
- Mental health issues
- Bereavements
- Retirement

There is a specific talking therapy called interpersonal therapy, where identifying and resolving interpersonal conflicts are thought to promote recovery [6].

Inform if the person is suitable or unsuitable for interpersonal therapy.

Do you think you would be motivated to engage in this therapy?

Family Therapy

Scenario

17-year-old Harriet Whitcombe has recently been diagnosed with schizophrenia. Her father Mr. Whitcombe is waiting to speak to you about family therapy.

Task

Explain family therapy.

Approach

Hello, I am Dr. _____. I am a psychiatrist. I understand your daughter has been diagnosed with schizophrenia and you are here to discuss family therapy.

Explain Family Therapy
- The psychological therapy is called family therapy.
- It sees the families as systems whereby the behaviour of one family member influences the behaviour of other family members.
- For example, you say something that is perceived in a poor light by your wife; this in turn affects her behaviour toward you, which results in you responding negatively toward her. This becomes a vicious cycle.
- Family therapy aims to break this cycle by understanding how the way we speak or behave might be perceived by others in the family.
- The therapy involves 12–16 weekly sessions with each session lasting around 1 h.
- All family members are encouraged to attend the sessions; however, the sessions can proceed with even a single family member.
- The therapy is delivered by a qualified therapist who will facilitate discussion between the family members.
- There will be a therapist in the next room who will be listening to the conversations and facilitating the discussion.
- High expressed emotions: When an individual has been diagnosed with schizophrenia, this affects the whole family. This can lead to the environment in the house becoming more emotional. Unknowingly, we can become excessively critical or protective of the family member. It is important to have a balanced approach.

The sessions will also include information on

- Recognising relapse signatures
- Problem-solving skills
- Communication skill training
- Social skill training [7]

Offer leaflets.

Station-Specific Points

Chunk and check.

Cognitive Behavioural Therapy

Scenario

Mr. George Blair is 40 years old with a diagnosis of depression and has been started on sertraline by the GP and referred to psychiatric services for cognitive behavioural therapy (CBT).

Task

Explain cognitive behavioural therapy.

Approach

Hello, I am Dr. _____. I am a psychiatrist. I understand you have been referred by the GP to discuss cognitive behavioural therapy or CBT.

- CBT is a form of talking therapy that looks at the thoughts, emotions and behaviour link.
- It is a simple and highly effective technique.
- It helps us examine our cognitions or thoughts.
- Identify errors in our thinking.
- Challenging negative thoughts.
- Replacing these negative thoughts with more realistic and positive thoughts.
- These negative thoughts can affect our emotions, which in turn adversely affects our behaviour.
- You will be requested to maintain a thoughts diary.
- You will also be requested to maintain an activity diary.

- The therapist will encourage the use of Socratic questioning.
- A qualified therapist works with the client to deliver the therapy.
- There will be a total of 8–20 sessions on a weekly basis with each session lasting around 1 h.
- It focuses on the here and now rather than past experiences.
- Strictly time-limited regular sessions.
- CBT can be practised at home with the homework that is allocated by the therapist.
- There may be some initial worsening of your symptoms as you explore your negative thoughts, but this will resolve over time [8].
- Psychoeducation.
- Leaflets.

Psychosocial Treatment for Schizophrenia

Scenario

Mr. Roger Aspen is a 40-year-old man with a diagnosis of schizophrenia and depression on aripiprazole and citalopram, who lives in a supported accommodation. The staff have requested a patient review to explain psychosocial interventions.

Task

Discuss the psychosocial interventions for schizophrenia.

Approach

Hello, I am Dr. ____. I am a psychiatrist. I am here to discuss the psychosocial treatment options for your condition.

How Would You Describe Your
- Mood
- Sleep
- Appetite
- Energy levels
- Interest in activities
- Motivation
- Concentration
- Hearing voices/seeing things
- Delusional beliefs
- Thought disorder

Risk Assessment
- Do you have any thoughts of suicide?
- Any suicidal plans?
- Any thoughts of deliberate self-harm [9]?

Social Support
- Family or friends that can offer support

Psychosocial Interventions
- Psychosocial interventions are based on the strength of the individual.
- They address the unique needs of the individual and empower him or her to better themselves.
- This is delivered using a structured programme.
- Psychoeducation about their condition.
- This involves the development of personal networks like natural supports with family/friends, self-help groups and various peer support initiatives.
- Family interventions.
- Life skill training—programmes to enhance practical life skills required to live independently like managing finances, self-care and developing domestic skills.
- Social skill training—to enhance social communication involving complex behaviours by using various techniques like modelling, role play and social reinforcement.
- Improving employment opportunities using pre-employment vocational training and supported employment.
- Cognitive behavioural therapy—a form of talking therapy is used to recognise errors in thinking, identify negative thoughts and replace with more realistic and positive thoughts.
- Cognitive rehabilitation—to improve social and work functioning by retraining of memory, attention and abstract problem-solving [10].

Cognitive Behavioural Therapy for Psychosis

Scenario

22-year-old Phoebe Sutherland had a psychotic episode for the first time 8 months ago. She was admitted to hospital and treated with quetiapine. She has regular follow-up with the community psychiatric nurse and is presently stable in her mental state.

Task

Develop a formulation, and briefly explain cognitive behavioural therapy for psychosis.

Approach

Hello, I am Dr. _____. I am a psychiatrist.

Presenting Complaints
- When did you first start having issues with your mental health?
- What were your symptoms?
- What were the circumstances that led to your admission?
- What medication you are on now? Do you take the medication regularly?
- Have you experienced any medication side effects?
- Brief MSE—enquire about mood, sleep, appetite anhedonia, hearing voices, seeing things, paranoia and suspicion.

Predisposing Factors
- Do you have a family history of mental health issues?
- Do you remember if your mother had any complications during her pregnancy with you?
- Do you remember if there were any problems at the time of delivery when you were born?
- When you think about your childhood, were there any difficult experiences like bullying, abuse or any other distressing incidents that you remember?

Precipitating Factors
- What was happening in your life around the time when you first started having mental health issues?
- Any stressful life events?
- Any major changes in your life?
- Any recreational drug use prior to hospital admission?

Perpetuating Factors
- Do you have any ongoing stressors?
- What are your thoughts about your diagnosis?
- What are your thoughts about medication?
- Any recreational drug use at present time?

Protective Factors
- What are your plans for the future?
- How is your relationship with your family?
- How do you view your illness?

Discuss a formulation using all the above information [11].

Explain CBT for Psychosis
- It is a form of talking therapy that is used in individuals who have unusual experiences that can be distressing. It looks at the thoughts, emotions and behaviour link.
- This therapy will help you explore alternate explanations for these experiences that are less distressing.
- You will be encouraged to use reality testing by challenging negative thoughts.
- Identification of clear, positive goals that are realistic and time limited [12].

Is this something you would be interested in?
Do you think you would be motivated enough to attend all the sessions?

Assess Cognitive Errors

Scenario

24-year-old Tom Shatner is a professional rugby player and has been struggling since he failed to score a goal in the recent match against a rival team.

Task

Assess cognitive errors.

Approach

Have a discussion with Tom to elicit the presence of the following cognitive errors:

- Catastrophising—thinking the worst
- Labelling—I am a loser
- Dichotomous thinking—nothing other than complete success or complete failure
- Minimisation—minimising previous achievements
- Magnification—maximise the fact that you did not score one goal
- Personalisation—it is my fault
- Overgeneralisation—I will never succeed again
- Arbitrary inference [13]

Enquire about recreational drug use and alcohol excess.

References

1. Semple D, Smyth R. Psychotherapy. Systematic desensitization. Oxford handbook of psychiatry. 3rd ed. Oxford University Press; 2017. p. 848.
2. Cowen P, Harrison P, Burns T. Psychological treatments. Exposure with response prevention. Shorter oxford textbook of psychiatry. 6th ed. Oxford University Press; 2012. p. 582.
3. Semple D, Smyth R. Chapter 2 Psychiatric assessment. History. Mental state examination. Oxford handbook of psychiatry. 3rd ed. Oxford University Press; 2017. p. 42–44.
4. Semple D, Smyth R. Psychotherapy. Defence mechanisms. Displacement. Oxford handbook of psychiatry. 3rd ed. Oxford University Press; 2017. p. 831.
5. Psychological treatments. Transference and countertransference. Shorter oxford textbook of psychiatry. 6th ed. Oxford University Press; 2012. p. 574.
6. Semple D, Smyth R. Interpersonal psychotherapy. Oxford handbook of psychiatry. 3rd ed. Oxford University Press; 2017. p. 854.
7. Cowen P, Harrison P, Burns T. Psychological treatments. Family therapy. Shorter oxford textbook of psychiatry. 6th ed. Oxford University Press; 2012. p. 596.
8. Semple D, Smyth R. Psychotherapy. Cognitive behavioural therapy. Oxford handbook of psychiatry. 3rd ed. Oxford University Press; 2017. p. 852.
9. Semple D, Smyth R. Psychiatric assessment. History. Oxford handbook of psychiatry. 3rd ed. Oxford University Press; 2017. p. 42.
10. Adams C, Wilson P. Psychosocial interventions for schizophrenia. BMJ Qual Saf. 2000;9:251.
11. Cowen P, Harrison P, Burns T. Assessment. Formulations. Shorter oxford textbook of psychiatry. 6th ed. Oxford University Press; 2012. p. 63.
12. Cowen P, Harrison P, Burns T. Psychological treatments. Cognitive-behaviour therapy for schizophrenia. Shorter oxford textbook of psychiatry. 6th ed. Oxford University Press; 2012. p. 588.
13. Semple D, Smyth R. Psychotherapy. Common types of cognitive errors. Oxford handbook of psychiatry. 3rd ed. Oxford University Press; 3rd. p. 851.

Sodium Valproate

Scenario

34-year-old Janet Reid has a diagnosis of bipolar affective disorder and has recently found out that she is 6 weeks pregnant. She has been on sodium valproate 800 mg for the last 10 years, and her mental health is stable. She has been referred by the GP to the outpatient psychiatry clinic.

Task

Explain the effects of sodium valproate in pregnancy.
  Address her ideas, concerns and expectations.
  Devise a management plan.

Approach

Hello, I am Dr. _____. I am a psychiatrist. I understand you are pregnant and taking sodium valproate.

Explain the Effects of Sodium Valproate
- In the first 3 months of pregnancy, the baby's organs develop and this is the most crucial period for baby's development.
- 10% of babies whose mothers are on sodium valproate during pregnancy will develop a birth defect, which means the baby does not develop properly. This is

---

All names and scenarios mentioned in this book are fictitious. Any resemblance to actual individuals or backgrounds is entirely conincidental.

© The Author(s), under exclusive license to Springer Nature Switzerland AG 2023
N. Sivaswamy, *Prepare for the MRCPsych CASC Exam*,
https://doi.org/10.1007/978-3-031-31019-5_9

in comparison to 2–3% of babies in mothers who are not on any medication in pregnancy.

- The baby can have spina bifida where the bones of the spine do not join up properly.
- The baby can also have other problems with the bones of the face and upper lip being split, bones of the hands and legs not developing properly and problems with the development of other organs like kidneys and heart.
- 30–40% of babies might have developmental delays—delays in walking and talking.
- There can also be poor language skills, memory problems and lower intelligence.
- There is an increased risk of the baby having conditions like attention deficit hyperactivity disorder and autism spectrum disorder.

Management
- Stop the sodium valproate immediately.
- Start antipsychotic medications that are relatively safe in pregnancy like olanzapine to ensure that your mental health does not deteriorate.
- Start folic acid tablet 5 mg, to be taken throughout pregnancy.
- We use a multidisciplinary team approach involving perinatal psychiatrists, obstetricians and midwives.
- Referral to perinatal psychiatry services.
- Liaising closely with the obstetric team to organise frequent ultrasound scans and specialist prenatal monitoring [1].
- It is important to emphasise that as you are 6 weeks pregnant, it is imperative to make a decision quickly.
- I will offer another appointment tomorrow, so you have time to think over all the information and convey your decision if you are unable to make up your mind right away.
- Leaflets.

Station-Specific Points

- Remember to chunk and check.
- Explain using jargon-free language.
- Respond to role player's questions, and deliver all information in a sensitive manner.

Lithium

Scenario

30-year-old Nancy Neil has a diagnosis of bipolar affective disorder and is planning a pregnancy. She is on lithium, and her mental health is stable. She has been referred by the GP to the outpatient psychiatry clinic.

Task

Explain the effects of lithium in pregnancy.
Address her queries.

Approach

Hello, I am Dr. _____. I am a psychiatrist. I understand you are planning to get pregnant, are presently taking lithium and have some queries about medication.

Explain the Effects of Lithium

- In the first 3 months of pregnancy, the baby's organs develop and this is the most crucial period for baby's development.
- Even when the mother has not taken any medication in pregnancy, about 2–3% of babies have a problem with the way their body develops, about 1% of babies have a heart problem and about 1 in 5 pregnancies end in miscarriage.
- There is a 1 in 10 chance of birth defects, that is, problems with the way the baby develops, if lithium is continued through the first 3 months of pregnancy.
- There is a heart problem called Ebstein's anomaly.
- The chance of the baby developing this condition is 1 in 1000 when lithium is continued during pregnancy. The chance of this condition in mothers who are not taking any medication in pregnancy is 1 in 20,000.
- Highest risk is 2–6 weeks after conception when most pregnancies are undetected.
- According to the National Institute for Health and Care Excellence guidelines, breastfeeding is not recommended on lithium as the levels in mother's body and breast milk are similar.

Management

There is the option to stop lithium or continue it, and we will discuss both.
Discontinuing lithium before getting pregnant:

- Reduce and stop the lithium.
- One option is to monitor mental health carefully without any medication during pregnancy.
- Another option is to start antipsychotic medication like olanzapine to ensure that your mental health does not deteriorate.

If lithium is continued during pregnancy:

- Monthly checks of lithium levels.
- From 36 weeks' pregnancy, weekly checks of lithium levels.
- Increasing doses of lithium may be required as pregnancy progresses.
- Lithium is stopped during active labour, and blood levels are checked within 12 h after delivery.

Delivery

- Delivery to happen in hospital, with mother and baby to remain in hospital and thoroughly checked to ensure well-being prior to discharge.
- If the mother goes into labour before due date, obstetricians will decide best management and inform mental health services, so we can provide ongoing support.
- The infant will be monitored for lithium-related issues—thyroid problems, floppiness, tiredness, heart problems and breathing difficulties.

General Points

- Referral to perinatal psychiatry services.
- Liaising closely with the obstetric team to organise frequent ultrasound scans and specialist prenatal monitoring [1].
- The mother and baby unit can be considered for admission if necessary.
- Leaflets.
- Offer another appointment to discuss any other queries they may have.

Post-partum Psychosis Management

Scenario

32-year-old Paula Newton has a diagnosis of bipolar affective disorder and is 35 weeks pregnant. She has had two previous episodes of post-partum psychosis and is now concerned about becoming unwell again. The current pregnancy was planned, and she came off lithium and quetiapine before getting pregnant. She has been referred by the GP to the outpatient psychiatry clinic. She prefers a medication option that will allow her to breastfeed her child.

Task

Address the patient's ideas, concerns and expectations.
Devise a management plan.

Approach

Hello, I am Dr. _____. I am a psychiatrist. I understand you are pregnant.

Explain

- The risk of developing post-partum psychosis in an individual with previous episodes is 1 in 5. As you have had two previous episodes, your risk is on the higher side.

- Since you are 35 weeks pregnant, you are sufficiently late in your pregnancy that lithium is unlikely to cause any problems in the development of the baby's body.
- However, according to the National Institute for Health and Care Excellence guidelines, lithium is not recommended in breastfeeding. This is because the amount of lithium in a mother's body is equivalent to the amount transferred to the baby through breast milk, and this is unsafe for the baby.
- Therefore, if you are interested in breastfeeding, we will consider other options, namely antipsychotic medication like olanzapine or quetiapine.
- Evidence states that antipsychotic medications are relatively safe in pregnancy.
- If a particular antipsychotic medication has worked well previously, we can consider starting that.
- There is a risk of gestational diabetes if the mother is on antipsychotic medication.
- We will use the lowest effective dose of medication.

Delivery
- Delivery to happen in hospital with specialist paediatric services available.
- Mother and baby to remain in hospital and thoroughly checked to ensure well-being prior to discharge.
- If the mother goes into labour before due date, obstetricians will decide best management and inform mental health services, so we can provide ongoing support.

Breastfeeding
- Time feeds around medication to avoid high levels of medication being passed through breast milk.
- Effects of antipsychotic—baby might be more restless with frequent crying.
- A mix of breastfeeding with bottle feeding will minimise these effects with the goal being to move on to exclusive bottle feeding [2].

Additional Points
- We will use a multidisciplinary team approach including obstetrician, midwife and perinatal psychiatrist.
- Referral to perinatal psychiatry services.
- If the mother becomes unwell, we have to consider admission to mother and baby unit.
- Psychoeducation to the family.
- Social support—support of partner and wider family members is very important.
- Leaflets.
- Future pregnancies—to be planned.

Station-Specific Points

- Admission to mother and baby unit if mother becomes unwell.
- Enquire about partner support.

Post-partum Depression Management

Scenario

21-year-old Amy MacDonald has a 2-week-old baby and has been diagnosed with postnatal depression. This is her first child. You are speaking to her husband Roger MacDonald.

Task

Explain the diagnosis and a management plan.

Approach

Hello, I am Dr. _____. I am a psychiatrist. I understand Mrs. MacDonald has recently been diagnosed with postnatal depression.

Explain Postnatal Depression
- Postnatal depression means becoming depressed after having the baby.
- 1 in 10 women have postnatal depression after childbirth.
- It usually occurs 1–3 months after having a baby.
- She can experience symptoms like being sad, having no energy, feeling hopeless, having suicidal thoughts and exaggerated concerns about baby.
- It is thought to be due to imbalance of chemicals in the brain.
- Risk factors—previous history of depression or postnatal depression, stressful events and poor partner/social support.
- Antidepressant medication—no antidepressant is completely safe in pregnancy or breastfeeding. However, medication like sertraline is preferable.
- Effects of antidepressants on baby—early delivery, low birth weight, irritability and breathing difficulties.
- Reassurance and support to your partner.
- Counselling or talking therapy.
- Marital counselling if necessary for marital issues.
- Psychoeducation for partner and family.
- Stress management techniques to prevent further episodes.
- Attend postnatal support groups.
- Information and advice on planning subsequent pregnancies.
- Ensure that the mother gets adequate sleep and has a healthy diet [3].

Genetics of Schizophrenia

Scenario

30-year-old Mrs. Shafa Ahmed has a diagnosis of schizophrenia and has been stable on olanzapine for 5 years. She has recently found out that she is pregnant and is concerned about the baby's chances of developing schizophrenia.

Task

Address her concerns.

Approach

Hello, I am Dr. ___. I am a psychiatrist. I understand you have some concerns. Would you like to tell me more?

- May I ask if anyone in the family other than you has schizophrenia?
- If one parent has schizophrenia, there is a 1 in 10 chance of the child developing the condition.
- In other words, approximately 1 in 10 people with schizophrenia has a parent with the illness. Therefore, there is a 9 in 10 chance that the baby will not develop this condition.
- To give you a bit of perspective in the general population, the risk of developing schizophrenia is 1%.
- It is usually caused by a combination of genetic and environmental factors.
- Genetic means it tends to run in families. However, there is no single reason for developing this condition, and it is usually a combination of several factors put together.
- Factors in pregnancy like viral infection in the mother, stress and a lack of oxygen to the baby have all been known to contribute to the risk of developing this condition.
- Cannabis use makes it six times more likely for an individual to develop schizophrenia.
- Amphetamine use has also been implicated.
- Other factors like stressful life events, family problems and adverse childhood experiences like abuse or deprivation are also implicated [4].
- Social support: May I ask if the father of the baby is supportive? With your consent, I can speak to your husband to explain the situation.
- I will refer to perinatal psychiatry services.

Opiate Dependence in Pregnancy

Scenario

27-year-old Emily Archibald has a history of heroin dependence. She has recently discovered that she is 5 weeks pregnant. She is concerned about the effects of heroin on her baby and is considering stopping heroin use. She is interested in discussing the options.

Task

Take a brief history of heroin dependence.

Explain the impact of heroin use on the developing baby and the management options to stop heroin use.

Approach

Hello, I am Dr. _____. I am a psychiatrist. I understand from the information I have that you are pregnant.

History of Presenting Complaint
- May I ask if it is a planned or unplanned pregnancy?
- Is the father of the baby supportive?
- How is your relationship with him?
- Do you have any other children? Do they reside with you?
- What drugs do you use?
- Have you ever used any other drugs—cannabis, cocaine or amphetamines?
- What drug are you using now?
- How often do you use this drug?
- How much of this drug do you take in a day?
- How much money do you spend in a day or week on drugs?
- How do you finance your drug use?
- What is your preferred route for drug use—oral, smoking or injected?

If injected:

- What sites do you use for injecting?
- Have you ever shared needles?
- Have you ever heard of the needle exchange programme?

May I ask if you use alcohol in excess?
Have you seen a psychiatrist in the past?

Brief Mental State Examination

Mood, sleep, appetite, anhedonia, hearing voices/seeing things that are not really there, suicidal thoughts and deliberate self-harm

Risk: sex for drugs and unprotected sexual intercourse while under the influence of drugs

Elicit the Core Symptoms of Opiate Dependence

- Do you crave for drugs sometimes?
- Do you find you have to take more amount to achieve the same effect?
- If you do not take drugs, do you experience withdrawal effects?

Additional Questions

- Have you ever had any treatment for the drug problem?
- Have you ever been in hospital for drug-related issues?
- Have you ever had any periods of abstinence?

Complications of Drug Use

- Have you had tests for hepatitis B, hepatitis C and HIV?
- Have you ever had any abscess, accidents, falls or head injury?
- Have you had any problems with the police—driving under the influence of drugs?
- Financial problems [5]?

Effects of Heroin Use on Baby

- Heroin itself does not cause problems in the way the baby's body develops.
- Heroin use in pregnancy may cause other problems for the baby like miscarriage, death in the womb and premature birth.
- The longer the duration of heroin use and greater the amount, the higher the risk it presents to the baby in the womb.

Treatment

1. The treatment for opiate dependence is methadone.
2. Methadone substitution can happen any time in pregnancy as it presents reduced risk for the baby than continued opiate use.
3. However, detoxification, that is, coming off the opiates completely using methadone, is undertaken only in the middle 3 months of pregnancy.
4. We avoid detoxification in the first 3 months of pregnancy due to risk of miscarriage and avoid the last 3 months of pregnancy due to risk of stillbirth.
5. The baby will be monitored carefully for withdrawal symptoms like irritability, loud crying, shakiness and sneezing.
6. Breastfeeding is allowed on methadone; however, the baby needs to be monitored for the side effects like being more sleepy.
7. Referral to substance misuse services.
8. Referral to perinatal psychiatry team.
9. Multidisciplinary team approach—obstetricians, psychiatrists, midwives and social work [6].

Station-Specific Points

- Social work involvement if the mother requires help and support.
- The baby remains with the mother unless there are significant concerns for safety of the baby.

Treatment-Resistant Depression and Pregnancy

Scenario

33-year-old Bethany Jamieson has a diagnosis of treatment-resistant depression. She currently takes fluoxetine 60 mg and lithium 400 mg. Her mental health has been stable on this combination. She is interested in planning a pregnancy and is concerned about the effect of medication on the baby when she gets pregnant.

Task

Discuss the effects of medication on the baby if she were to get pregnant and answer her queries.

Approach

Hello, I am Dr. _____. I am a psychiatrist. I understand you are planning a pregnancy and would like to discuss various management options regarding medication.

Even when the mother has not taken any medication:

- About 2–3 in 100 babies have a birth defect, which is a problem in the way baby's body develops.
- About 1 in 100 babies has a heart defect, which is a problem in the way the baby's heart develops.
- About 1 in 5 pregnancies ends in miscarriage.

Lithium
- In the first 3 months of pregnancy, the baby's organs develop, and this is the most crucial period for baby's development.
- There is a problem with the development of the heart called Ebstein's anomaly. The risk of developing this condition if lithium is continued in pregnancy is 1 in 1000 babies. When the mother is not on medication in pregnancy, the chance of developing this condition is 1 in 20,000 babies [7].

- Highest risk is 2–6 weeks after conception when most pregnancies are undetected.
- Breastfeeding is not recommended on lithium as the levels in the mother's blood and breast milk are similar.
- In the infant, lithium toxicity presents as floppiness, tiredness, heart problems and breathing difficulties.
- The birth must take place in a hospital.

If lithium is continued during pregnancy:

- Monthly checks of lithium levels.
- From 36 weeks' pregnancy, weekly checks of lithium levels.
- Increasing doses may be required as pregnancy progresses.
- Lithium is stopped during labour and checked within 12–24 h after delivery. The dose is adjusted and then checked again in 5–7 days [1].

Antidepressant
- Fluoxetine is one of the antidepressants that is relatively safe; however, sertraline is preferable.
- Ideally, we use the lowest effective dose and avoid medication that remains in the body for a long time, which is the reason we would prefer not to use fluoxetine.
- Effects of antidepressants on baby—preterm delivery, low birth weight, irritability and breathing difficulties.
- Breastfeeding is thought to be relatively safe on antidepressant medication [8].

Management
- Partner and family support are very important.
- We use a multidisciplinary team approach involving perinatal psychiatrists, obstetricians and midwives.
- Referral to perinatal psychiatry services.
- Liaising closely with the obstetric team to organise frequent ultrasound scans and specialist prenatal monitoring [1].

Station-Specific Points

- Chunk and check.
- Offer leaflets.
- Offer another appointment to discuss any further queries they may have.

References

1. Taylor DM, Barnes T, Young A. Bipolar illness during pregnancy and postpartum. Treatment with mood stabilisers. The Maudsley prescribing guidelines in psychiatry. 14th ed. Wiley Blackwell; 2021. p. 689.
2. Taylor DM, Barnes T, Young A. Psychosis during pregnancy and postpartum. The Maudsley prescribing guidelines in psychiatry. 14th ed. Wiley Blackwell; 2021. p. 681.
3. Taylor DM, Barnes T, Young A. Pregnancy and breastfeeding. Depression during pregnancy and postpartum. The Maudsley prescribing guidelines in psychiatry. 14th ed. Wiley Blackwell; 2021. p. 685.
4. Royal College of Psychiatrists. Schizophrenia: for parents and carers. Royal College of Psychiatrists. https://www.rcpsych.ac.uk/mental-health/parents-and-young-people/information-for-parents-and-carers/schizophrenia-for-parents. Accessed November 2015.
5. Semple D, Smyth R. Substance misuse. Assessment of the drug user. Oxford handbook of psychiatry. 3rd ed. Oxford University Press; 2017. p. 592.
6. National Institute for Health and Care Excellence. Opioid dependence: managing special circumstances. 2022. https://cks.nice.org.uk/topics/opioid-dependence/management/managing-special-circumstances/. Accessed April.
7. Royal College of Psychiatrists London. Lithium in pregnancy and breastfeeding. https://www.rcpsych.ac.uk/mental-health/treatments-and-wellbeing/lithium-in-pregnancy-and-breastfeeding.
8. Taylor DM, Barnes T, Young A. Depression during pregnancy and postpartum. The Maudsley prescribing guidelines in psychiatry. 14th ed. Wiley Blackwell; 2021. p. 685.

Explanations

Lithium Augmentation

Scenario

44-year-old Jackson Cartwright is an inpatient in the psychiatric ward following a diagnosis of moderate-to-severe depression. He has been started on fluoxetine with a partial response. At the team meeting, it was decided to augment with lithium.

Task

Explain lithium augmentation.
Address the patient's ideas, concerns and expectations.

Approach

Hello, I am Dr. ___. I am a psychiatrist. I understand you have a diagnosis of depression. At the team meeting today, the decision was made to augment your existing medication with lithium.

Lithium
- Lithium is a chemical that occurs naturally in food and water.
- It is used as a mood stabiliser to treat and control mood disorders like depression.
- It is also used to boost or augment the effect of antidepressant medication when they do not work well on their own.

All names and scenarios mentioned in this book are fictitious. Any resemblance to actual individuals or backgrounds is entirely conincidental.

© The Author(s), under exclusive license to Springer Nature
Switzerland AG 2023
N. Sivaswamy, *Prepare for the MRCPsych CASC Exam*,
https://doi.org/10.1007/978-3-031-31019-5_10

Side Effects

Short Term

- Feeling sick
- Metallic taste in mouth
- Loose stools
- Increased thirst
- Passing urine frequently
- Trembling of hands
- Muscle aches
- Dry mouth

Long Term

- Weight gain
- Changes in kidney function
- Changes in thyroid function
- Shaky hands
- Skin rash
- Worsen pre-existing skin conditions like acne or psoriasis

Investigations

- Prior to starting lithium, we will perform blood tests including kidney function and thyroid function and do a tracing of your heart.
- We will also check the lithium level in your blood initially on a weekly basis. This is to ascertain the level of lithium that remains within the treatment range.

Treatment Range

- Lithium has to be within a particular level called the treatment range usually 0.6–0.8 to be effective.
- If it is too low, it will be ineffective, and if it is too high it can lead to toxicity.
- As previously mentioned, the lithium level is checked weekly; then once stable, it can be checked monthly and thereafter every few months.

Toxicity

When the level of lithium increases above the treatment range, the individual can experience:

- Vomiting
- Persistent loose stools
- Slurred speech
- Confusion
- Fits

This is an emergency, so please contact us immediately if you experience any of these symptoms.

Interactions

- Lithium can interact with painkillers and medication that lowers blood pressure.
- Please inform your doctor that you are on lithium when starting any new medication [1].

Station-Specific Points

- Lithium treatment pack
- Leaflets
- Remember to chunk and check

Clozapine

Scenario

39-year-old Marvin Dunlop has recently received a diagnosis of treatment-resistant psychosis, and the decision has been made by the treating team to start on clozapine.

Task

Explain the decision to start clozapine and details of the medication.

Approach

I am Dr. ___. I am a psychiatrist. I understand you have recently received a diagnosis of treatment-resistant schizophrenia. The treating team has made the decision to start a new medication called clozapine.

Clozapine

- It is a highly effective medication that balances the levels of a chemical called dopamine in the brain.
- 6 out of 10 patients benefit from taking clozapine.
- It is prescribed according to the National Institute for Health and Care Excellence guidelines and is not given earlier in the treatment process as it has some side effects that require regular monitoring.

Side Effects

- Feeling more sleepy
- Increased saliva production
- Weight gain
- Constipation
- Changes in blood pressure

There are some side effects that we are concerned about and closely monitor for:

- Agranulocytosis—the body has specific cells that help us fight germs that enter our body. In people who take clozapine, the number of these cells decreases.
- This can occur in 2–3 of every 10 patients on clozapine.
- This increases the risk of becoming unwell. Therefore, we advise that if you ever develop a sore throat or fever, contact us immediately.
- Myocarditis—this medication can affect the muscles of the heart.

Investigations
- Prior to starting clozapine, we will perform blood tests checking your blood counts, kidney function and liver function and do a tracing of your heart.

Monitoring
- We will perform the above tests on a weekly basis for 18 weeks.
- Then every second week until the end of the first year of treatment with clozapine.
- Following this, if all remains well, the tests will be on a monthly basis for as long as you remain on clozapine.

Additional Points
- It will be started at a small dose and slowly increased.
- Smoking changes the amount of clozapine available in the body; therefore, higher doses may be required.
- If you decrease the number of cigarettes or stop smoking, please do let us know, so we can monitor and adjust the dose of clozapine accordingly [2].
- Leaflets

Station-Specific Points

- Avoid using jargon.
- Allow time for the role player to ask questions.
- Chunk and check.

Electroconvulsive Therapy

Scenario

39-year-old Dominic Stevenson was diagnosed with severe depression, and the consultant has decided to start electroconvulsive therapy (ECT). His wife Eugenia Stevenson is aware of this decision and is waiting to speak to you.

Task

Explain electroconvulsive therapy.

Approach

Hello, I am Dr. _____. I am a psychiatrist.

Explain Electroconvulsive Therapy
- A small controlled current is used to induce a brief fit lasting usually no more than 30 s.
- The procedure takes place in a special treatment room with an anaesthetist who inserts a small needle into your arm and administers general anaesthesia so the person will be asleep during the entire procedure.
- A medication will be given to relax your muscles and reduce body movements during the procedure.
- The small controlled electric current will be delivered by placing two pads on either side of your head.
- After the procedure, the person will wake up a short while later in the recovery room, supervised and monitored by staff until ready to return to ward or leave the treatment room.
- A course of electroconvulsive therapy is usually 6–12 sessions in total with a session twice a week.
- You will be requested to provide written consent prior to the procedure.
- You can withdraw consent at any time.

Explain Side Effects
Short Term
- Headaches
- Feeling sleepy

These side effects usually settle in a few hours.

Long Term
- Memory problems are usually short term but can be long term.
- If this continues to be an issue, we can consider unilateral electroconvulsive therapy, which means the pad will be applied to only one side of the head.

Prior to Starting the Electroconvulsive Therapy
The individual will have:

- Blood tests
- Electrical tracing of the heart

- Detailed physical examination
- Assessment by the anaesthetist [3]

  Leaflets

Station-Specific Points

- Avoid using jargon.
- Allow time for the role player to ask questions.
- Chunk and check.

Antidementia Medication

Scenario

80-year-old Ewen Mills was recently diagnosed with Alzheimer's dementia, and the plan is to start on medication. His wife Patricia Mills is waiting to speak to you.

Task

Explain the medication for dementia.

Approach

Hello, I am Dr. _____. I am a psychiatrist.

Explain Antidementia Medication
- In Alzheimer's dementia, there is a decrease of a chemical in the brain called acetylcholine which is responsible for memory.
- The medication increases levels of this chemical in the brain to stabilise memory and functioning.
- The medications available are donepezil, galantamine and rivastigmine.
- All three medication are quite similar. However, donepezil has the advantage of once-daily administration.
- This medication is not addictive.
- We start the medication at the lowest dose and slowly increase the dose.
- Unfortunately, this is not a cure; however, it will slow down the progress of the condition.

Explain Side Effects
- Feeling sick
- Vomiting
- Muscle aches
- Retaining urine
- Change how fast the heart beats

Investigations

Prior to starting the medication, we will take a detailed medical history especially looking for:

- Heart problems
- Stomach ulcers
- Asthma

We will perform blood tests checking:

- Full blood count
- Kidney function
- Liver function
- Thyroid function

Perform a tracing of your heart.

Monitoring
- We will perform regular tests of memory to check response to medication.
- We monitor the person regularly for side effects and have frequent reviews every 3–6 months [4].

Leaflets

Genetics in Alzheimer's Dementia

Scenario

88-year-old Colin Duguid has recently been diagnosed with dementia. His daughter 50-year-old Mrs. Penelope Taylor is waiting to speak to you as she is concerned about her chances of developing this condition.

Task

Address her ideas and concerns.

Approach

I am Dr. ___. I am a psychiatrist.

- It is difficult to say for certain who will develop the condition.
- The risk of inheriting the disorder is 3–4 times higher in first-degree relatives.
- In other words, there is a 15–19% chance in first-degree relatives versus 5% in the general population.
- Only 1% of all cases of Alzheimer's dementia are genetic and passed from generation to generation.
- If there is a genetic predisposition, that is, if it runs in families, the condition tends to begin at an earlier age, in the 40s or 50s.

Risk Factors for Developing Alzheimer's Dementia
- Increasing age is the primary risk factor.
- 10% of people over the age of 65 years and 40% over the age of 85 years will have Alzheimer's dementia.
- History of head injury.
- Previous history of depression.
- Less than 8 years of educational attainment.
- Having Down's syndrome.
- Physical health issues like high blood pressure, diabetes and high cholesterol can also contribute.

Testing
- Genes are proteins that are a base of hereditary.
- There is a gene called apolipoprotein E that has been shown to play a role in the development of Alzheimer's dementia.
- Testing for the gene is not recommended as it is not found in all cases of dementia, and this gene can also be found in patients without dementia.
- Therefore, testing for this gene is not diagnostic and has no predictive value [5].

Additional Points
- There is no evidence that smoking protects against Alzheimer's dementia.
- Maintain a good balanced diet and regular exercise, stop smoking and limit alcohol consumption.
- Mental activity—reading, sudoku and puzzles.
- Social activity—visiting family and friends and volunteering.

Electrocardiogram: Complete Heart Block

Scenario

40-year-old James Melville had a routine electrocardiogram (ECG) done as part of investigations as he is on amitriptyline. The electrocardiogram is showing some abnormalities.

Task

Explain the findings of the electrocardiogram, and devise a management plan.

Approach

Hello, I am Dr. _____. I am a psychiatrist. I understand you have had an electrocardiogram, and we are here to discuss the findings.

May I ask a few questions please before I go on to discuss the findings of the electrocardiogram?

- Do you have any chest pain?

Do You Have Any Shortness of Breath?
- Do you have any dizziness?
- Have you noticed any swelling of your ankles?
- Do you smoke?
- Do you think you are overweight?

Medical History
- May I ask if you have diabetes or high blood sugar?
- Do you have high blood pressure?
- Do you have increased cholesterol or unhealthy fats in your body?
- Do you have any heart problems?
- Have you previously had heart attack or stroke?

Family History
Any family history of heart problems or stroke?

Explain the Electrocardiogram
- The heart is a large pump made of specialised muscles with electrical messages telling it how to work.
- You have just had an electrocardiogram, which is an electrical recording of your heart [6].

Complete Heart Block

- The heart beats in a cycle with the upper chamber contracting to push the blood out and then the lower chamber doing the same.
- The electrical messages telling the heart when to pump are not working well, so the messages are not getting through.
- Therefore, the heart does not beat in this regular cycle and not enough blood is being pumped around the body.
- This can lead to sudden collapse and can be life-threatening.

Management

1. I will discuss with cardiology department urgently.
2. I will refer to them for transcutaneous pacing—a procedure which will help your heart beat in a regular manner.
3. I will arrange for you to go to the accident and emergency department immediately [7].

Electrocardiogram: QT Prolongation

Scenario

41-year-old Cameron Patters had a routine electrocardiogram done as part of investigations as he is on clozapine. The electrocardiogram is showing some abnormalities.

Task

Explain the findings of the electrocardiogram, and devise a management plan.

Approach

Hello, I am Dr. _____. I am a psychiatrist. I understand you have had an electrocardiogram, and we are here to discuss the findings.

May I ask a few questions please before I go on to discuss the findings of the electrocardiogram?

- Do you have any chest pain?
- Do you have any shortness of breath?
- Do you have any dizziness?
- Have you noticed any swelling of your ankles?
- Do you smoke?
- Do you think you are overweight?

Medical History
- May I ask if you have diabetes or high blood sugars?
- Do you have high blood pressure?
- Do you have increased cholesterol or unhealthy fats in your body?
- Do you have any heart problems?
- Have you previously had heart attack or stroke?

Family History
Any family history of heart problems or stroke?

Explain the Electrocardiogram
- The heart is a large pump made of specialised muscles with electrical messages telling it how to work.
- You have just had an electrocardiogram, which is an electrical recording of your heart [6].

QTc Prolongation
- The electrical messages telling your heart how to pump are delayed. This is serious and can be life-threatening.

Management
- QTc less than 500—repeat electrocardiogram, discuss with cardiology, consider reducing antipsychotic dose or switch to aripiprazole.
- QTc greater than 500—stop the antipsychotic, repeat electrocardiogram, get an immediate cardiology opinion and switch to aripiprazole [8].

Electrocardiogram: Myocardial Infarction

Scenario

53-year-old Steven Annand had a routine electrocardiogram (ECG) done as part of investigations as he is on clozapine. The electrocardiogram is showing some abnormalities.

Task

Explain the findings of the electrocardiogram, and devise a management plan.

Approach

Hello, I am Dr. _____. I am a psychiatrist. I understand you have had an electrocardiogram and are here to discuss the findings.

May I ask a few questions please before I go on to discuss the findings of the electrocardiogram?

- Do you have any chest pain?
- Do you have any shortness of breath?
- Do you have any dizziness?
- Have you noticed any swelling of your ankles?
- Do you smoke?
- Do you think you are overweight?

Medical History
- May I ask if you have diabetes or high blood sugars?
- Do you have high blood pressure?
- Do you have increased cholesterol or unhealthy fats in your body?
- Do you have any heart problems?
- Have you previously had heart attack or stroke?

Family History
Any family history of heart problems or stroke?

Explain the Electrocardiogram
- The heart is a large pump made of specialised muscles with electrical messages telling it how to work.
- You have just had an electrocardiogram, which is an electrical recording of your heart [6].

Silent Myocardial Infarction
- You are having a heart attack.
- Because you have no symptoms like chest pain and shortness of breath, it is called silent myocardial infarction or silent heart attack.
- This is more common in people with diabetes.
- It happens because a blood vessel in the heart becomes blocked, thus stopping blood flow to parts of the heart.
- This causes the muscle in that area to die and not work properly.

Management
- This is a medical emergency.
- I will immediately arrange to send you to the accident and emergency department.
- Psychiatric medication has no role in causing this.
- Long-term treatment is modification of risk factors [9].

Depot Medication

Scenario

25-year-old Vincent Fairchild has a diagnosis of schizophrenia and is non-compliant with his prescribed aripiprazole. His treating team has made the decision to start him on depot medication. He has given consent for you to speak to his mother.

Task

Speak to his mother Mrs. Rosie Fairchild. Explain the decision to start on depot medication and answer her questions.

Approach

Hello, I am Dr. _____. I am a psychiatrist. I understand the team has decided to start Vincent on depot medication. I am here to explain this in detail and answer any queries you may have.

Q1. What is depot medication?

A1. Depot is an injectable form of antipsychotic medication that is used to treat conditions like schizophrenia.

Q2. How does this medication work?

A2. It works the same way as the tablet form of antipsychotic medication and balances the levels of chemical called dopamine in the brain that is altered in schizophrenia.

Q3. How is it started?

A3. Initially, a small dose is started to test for any side effects and if all goes well it will be given regularly.

Q4. How often should it be given?

A4. Depending on the antipsychotic medication, the depot needs to be administered every week, 2 weeks, 4 weeks or 3 months. The decision on which antipsychotic to start will be based on the best interest of the individual.

Q5. How is it given?

A5. The injection is usually administered in the gluteal muscle in the buttock. The injection can be administered by trained staff at the mental health unit; the GP surgery or a community psychiatric nurse can administer it at your home.

Q6. What are the side effects?

A6. The localised effects related to the injection are mild pain and swelling that will settle quickly. The injection site is alternated to reduce these effects. Other side effects are similar to the tablet form such as weight gain and feeling more drowsy.

Q7. What are the benefits?

A7. The individual does not have to remember to take the medication as it is administered 1–4 weeks rather than daily.

Q8. What if he misses a dose?

A8. There is an increased risk of developing mental health issues again if he does not get his medication as prescribed [10].

References

1. British National Formulary. Lithium carbonate. 2021. https://bnf.nice.org.uk/drug/lithium-carbonate.html#sideEffects.

2. Electronic Medicines Compendium (EMC). Clozaril 100 mg tablets. https://www.medicines.org.uk/emc/product/10290/smpc.

3. Royal College of Psychiatrists, Committee on ECT and Related Treatments. Statement on Electroconvulsive Therapy (ECT). Position statement CERT01/17. Statement on Electroconvulsive Therapy (ECT). https://www.rcpsych.ac.uk/docs/default-source/about-us/who-we-are/electroconvulsive-therapy%2D%2D-ect-ctee-statement-feb17.pdf?sfvrsn=2f4a94f9_2. Accessed February 2017.

4. National Institute for Health and Care Excellence. Dementia: assessment, management and support for people living with dementia and their carers NICE guideline [NG97]. https://www.nice.org.uk/guidance/NG97/chapter/Recommendations#pharmacological-management-of-alzheimers-disease. Accessed 20 June 2018.

5. Alzheimer's Society. Genetics of dementia. Factsheet 405LP. https://www.alzheimers.org.uk/sites/default/files/pdf/factsheet_genetics_of_dementia.pdf. Accessed June 2021.

6. Tidy C. Cardiovascular history and examination. https://patient.info/doctor/cardiovascular-history-and-examination. Accessed February 2022.

7. Knabben V, Chhabra L, Slane M. Third-degree atrioventricular block. 2022. https://www.ncbi.nlm.nih.gov/books/NBK545199/. Accessed August.

8. Taylor DM, Barnes T, Young A. Schizophrenia and related psychoses. Antipsychotic adverse effects. ECG changes-QT prolongation. The Maudsley prescribing guidelines in psychiatry. 14th ed. Wiley Blackwell; 2021. p. 141.

9. Gul Z, Makaryus AN. Silent myocardial ischemia. 2022. https://www.ncbi.nlm.nih.gov/books/NBK536915/. Accessed August.

10. Royal College of Psychiatrists. Depot medication. https://www.rcpsych.ac.uk/mental-health/treatments-and-wellbeing/depot-medication.

Capacity Assessment

Financial Capacity Assessment

Scenario

46-year-old Ethan Thompson has been referred by his GP after his support worker expressed concerns that Ethan had not paid his landlord rent for the last 6 months.

Task

Assess financial capacity.

Approach

Hello, I am Dr. _____. I am a psychiatrist. I understand you have not paid your rent, and I am going to ask you a few questions around that please.

Finances
- May I ask how long you have not paid your rent?
- Why have you not paid your rent?
- Have you ever been in arrears on your rent before?
- May I ask what your source of income is?
- How much do you receive in a week/month?
- How do you manage your expenses?
- Do you have any difficulty paying your bills on time?

All names and scenarios mentioned in this book are fictitious. Any resemblance to actual individuals or backgrounds is entirely conincidental.

© The Author(s), under exclusive license to Springer Nature Switzerland AG 2023

N. Sivaswamy, *Prepare for the MRCPsych CASC Exam*, https://doi.org/10.1007/978-3-031-31019-5_11

- Are there arrears on other bills?
- Do you have a bank account?
- Can you tell me the different ways of depositing or withdrawing money from the bank—ATM, debit card or cheque?
- Have you heard of direct debit payments?
- If someone asks for your ATM debit card pin number, would you give it to them?
- If someone asks for your bank account details, would you share it with them?
- Would you be able to identify different denomination of notes?
- For example, you go to a shop and buy a loaf of bread that costs 2 pounds and you give the cashier a 10-pound note. How much change would you expect?
- What are the benefits of paying your rent on time?
- What are the risks of not paying your rent on time?
- We discussed the different ways of withdrawing money from the bank—can you tell me what they are?
- What do you intend to do about the arrears on rent that you have accumulated?

Brief Mental State Examination

- Ask about mood, sleep, appetite, anhedonia, psychosis, anxiety, suicidal thoughts and thoughts of harming the landlord.
- Have you seen a psychiatrist before? Do you have a psychiatric diagnosis?
- Are you on any regular medication? Do you take it as prescribed?
- From our discussion today, it appears that you do have capacity/lack capacity to make decisions about your finances. I will inform your GP [1].

Station-Specific Points

- Complete a financial capacity assessment.
- Do a brief mental state examination.
- Convey to the role player if they have or lack capacity.

Financial Capacity Assessment with Hoarding

Scenario

56-year-old James Baron has been referred to psychiatric services after his support worker raised concerns with the GP that James was hoarding things in his flat and had not paid the landlord rent for 2 months.

Task

Assess financial capacity.

Approach

Hello, I am Dr. ___. I am a psychiatrist. I understand you have not paid your rent, and I am going to ask you a few questions around that please.

Finances
- May I ask how long you have not paid your rent?
- Why have you not paid your rent?
- Have you ever been in arrears on your rent before?
- May I ask what your source of income is?
- How much do you receive in a week/month?
- How do you manage your expenses?
- Do you have any difficulty paying your bills on time?
- Are there arrears on other bills?
- Do you have a bank account?
- Can you tell me the different ways of depositing or withdrawing money from the bank—ATM, debit card or cheque?
- Have you heard of direct debit payments?
- If someone asks for your ATM debit card pin number, would you give it to them?
- If someone asks for your bank account details, would you share it with them?
- Would you be able to identify different denominations of notes?
- For example, you go to a shop and buy a loaf of bread that costs 2 pounds and you give the cashier a 10-pound note. How much change would you expect?
- We discussed the different ways of withdrawing money from the bank—can you tell me what they are?
- What are the benefits of paying your rent on time?
- What are the risks of not paying your rent on time?
- What do you intend to do about the arrears on rent that you have?

Brief Mental State Examination
- Ask about mood, sleep, appetite, anhedonia, psychosis, anxiety, suicidal thoughts and thoughts of harming the landlord.
- I understand you are collecting some items in your flat—what are these, and why do you collect them?
- Has anyone ever expressed concerns that these items may pose a health and safety hazard?
- Are any of these items flammable?
- Have you ever tripped on or fallen over these items?
- Have you seen a psychiatrist before? Do you have a psychiatric diagnosis?
- Are you on any regular medication? Do you take it as prescribed?
- From our discussion today, it appears that you do have capacity/lack capacity to make decisions about your finances. I will inform your GP [1].

Station-Specific Points

- Complete a financial capacity assessment.
- Do a brief mental state examination.
- Ask queries around the hoarding behaviour, and do a focused risk assessment.
- Convey to the role player if they have or lack capacity.

Financial Capacity Assessment and Delusions of Grandeur

Scenario

44-year-old Catherine Beason has been referred by his GP after his support worker expressed concerns that she had not paid the landlord rent for the last 3 months. Catherine also mentioned to the support worker that she was a distant relative of the royal family.

Task

Assess financial capacity.

Approach

Hello, I am Dr. _____. I am a psychiatrist. I understand you have not paid your rent, and I am going to ask you a few questions around that please.

Finances
- May I ask how long you have not paid your rent?
- Why have you not paid your rent?
- Have you ever been in arrears on your rent before?
- May I ask what your source of income is?
- How much do you receive in a week/month?
- How do you manage your expenses?
- Do you have any difficulty paying your bills on time?
- Are there arrears on other bills?
- Do you have a bank account?
- Can you tell me the different ways of depositing and withdrawing money from the bank—ATM, debit card or cheque?
- Have you heard of direct debit payments?
- If someone asks for your ATM debit card pin number, would you give it to them?
- If someone asks for your bank account details, would you share it with them?
- Would you be able to identify different denominations of notes?

- For example, you go to a shop and buy a loaf of bread that costs 2 pounds and you give the cashier a 10-pound note. How much change would you expect?
- We discussed the different ways of withdrawing money from the bank—can you tell me what they are?
- What are the benefits of paying your rent on time?
- What are the risks of not paying your rent on time?
- What do you intend to do about the arrears on rent that you have?

Brief Mental State Examination

- Ask about mood, sleep, appetite, anhedonia, psychosis, anxiety, suicidal thoughts and thoughts of harming the landlord.
- Explore the delusional beliefs and the association with not paying the rent.
- Specifically ask if she hears voices telling them not to pay the rent.
- Assess fixity and conviction of the delusional beliefs.
- Have you seen a psychiatrist before? Do you have a psychiatric diagnosis?
- Are you on any regular medication? Do you take it as prescribed?
- From our discussion today, it appears that you do have capacity/lack capacity to make decisions about your finances [1].

Station-Specific Points

- Complete a thorough financial capacity assessment.
- Do a brief mental state examination.
- Explore any delusions about being related to royalty.
- Convey to the role player if they have or lack capacity.

Medical Capacity Assessment Surgical Closure of Laceration

Scenario

39-year-old Jacob Wiseman has a diagnosis of borderline personality disorder and cut his neck following an argument with his boyfriend. He was reviewed by the surgeons in the hospital who have advised that the wound is deep, with no damage to underlying structures, and required to be closed under general anaesthesia. Jacob is refusing treatment and asking to return home.

Task

Assess medical capacity.

Approach

Hello, I am Dr. _____. I am a psychiatrist. I understand you have cut your neck.

- May I ask why you cut your neck?
- Have you done anything like this before?
- Are you on any medication?
- Do you take it as prescribed?

Brief Mental State Examination
- Mood, sleep, appetite, anhedonia, hearing voices and seeing things.
- Do you hear voices telling you to cut your neck?
- Do you still have thoughts of cutting your neck?
- Do you have any thoughts of suicide?
- Do you have any thoughts of self-harm?

Capacity
- What is your understanding of what the surgeons have advised?
- The risks of not having the procedure—scarring and infection.
- Have you been told that taking antibiotics would reduce your risk of infection?
- What are the benefits of having the procedure?
- May I ask why you do not want to have the procedure?
- May I clarify if there is any part of the procedure that you are unclear about and would like me to explain?
- Please could you tell me again what the risks are of not having the procedure?
- What is your decision about the procedure?
- From our discussion today, it appears that you do have capacity/lack capacity to make decisions about your medical treatment [2].

Station-Specific Points

- Complete a medical capacity assessment.
- Do a brief mental state examination.
- Convey to the role player if they have or lack capacity.

Medical Capacity Assessment: Endoscopy

Scenario

54-year-old Gregory Buchanan had an episode of haematemesis and has been reviewed by the gastroenterologists who advised endoscopy. He is refusing the procedure. He has a diagnosis of schizophrenia, and his community psychiatric nurse has also expressed concerns that he has recently been non-compliant with medication.

Task

Assess medical capacity.

Approach

Hello, I am Dr. ____. I am a psychiatrist. I understand you are refusing the endoscopy as advised by the doctors.

- May I ask why you are refusing the procedure?
- What medication are you on?
- I understand you have not been taking your medication. Why is that?

Brief Mental State Examination
- Mood, sleep, appetite, anhedonia, hearing voices, seeing things and suicidal thoughts
- Do you hear voices telling you not to have the procedure?
- Do you have any thoughts of suicide or self-harm?

Capacity
- What is your understanding of the procedure as explained by the surgeons?
- The risks of not having the procedure—further bleeding and ongoing blood loss, which can even be fatal.
- What are the benefits of having the procedure?
- May I ask why you do not want to have the procedure?
- May I clarify if there is any part of the procedure that you are unclear about and would like me to explain.
- Please could you tell me again what the risks are of not having the procedure?
- What is your decision about the procedure?
- From our discussion today, it appears that you do have capacity/lack capacity to make decisions about your treatment [2].

Station-Specific Points

- Complete a medical capacity assessment.
- Do a brief mental state examination.
- Convey to the role player if they have or lack capacity.

Social Care Capacity Assessment

Scenario

72-year-old Harrison Muir had a stroke and was recently discharged following a prolonged hospital stay after a stroke. Arrangements have been made for a care package, which he is declining to accept.

Task

Assess capacity to refuse the social care package.

Approach

Hello, I am Dr. ____. I am a psychiatrist. I understand you are declining to accept the care package.

- May I ask why you are refusing the package?
- Are you on any medication?
- Do you take it as prescribed?
- How is your memory?
- What kind of social support do you have?

Brief Mental State Examination
- Mood, sleep, appetite, anhedonia, hearing voices and seeing things
- Do you hear voices telling you to decline the care package?
- Do you have any thoughts of suicide or self-harm?

Capacity
- What is your understanding of the care package?
- What are the risks of declining the care package?
- What are the benefits of accepting the care package?
- May I clarify if there is any particular aspect of the care package that is unclear to you or you are not comfortable with?
- I can try and speak to your treating team to consider altering the care package if that is helpful.
- Please could you tell me again what the risks are of declining the care package?
- What is your decision about the package?
- From our discussion today, it appears that you do have capacity/lack capacity to make decisions about your social care package. I will inform your treating team [2].

Station-Specific Points

- Do a brief mental state examination.
- Convey to the role player if they have or lack capacity.

References

1. Fitch C, Chaplin R, Trend C, Collard S. Debt and mental health: the role of psychiatrists. Adv Psychiatr Treat. 2007;13:194.
2. Scottish Government. Adults with incapacity: guide to assessing capacity. https://www.gov. scot/publications/adults-incapacity-scotland-act-2000-communication-assessing-capacity-guide-social-work-health-care-staff/pages/2/. Accessed 1 Feb 2008.

Examination

Schizophrenia

Scenario

38-year-old Belinda Burke has been referred by the GP as she was hearing voices.

Task

Perform a mental state examination.

Approach

Hello, I am Dr. _____. I am a psychiatrist. I understand you have been referred by the GP due to some concerns.

Please tell me more about the voices you are hearing.

Hallucinations

Auditory hallucinations

- How many voices do you hear?
- Do you recognise them?
- Do they talk to you directly?
- Do they talk among themselves about you?
- Do they give you instructions?
- What do they say?

All names and scenarios mentioned in this book are fictitious. Any resemblance to actual individuals or backgrounds is entirely conincidental.

© The Author(s), under exclusive license to Springer Nature Switzerland AG 2023

N. Sivaswamy, *Prepare for the MRCPsych CASC Exam*, https://doi.org/10.1007/978-3-031-31019-5_12

- Do you obey them?
- Do they give a running commentary?
- Do you hear the voices in your head or from outside?

Visual hallucinations
Olfactory hallucinations
Gustatory hallucinations
Tactile hallucinations

Comment on Appearance and Behaviour
Depressive Symptoms
- Mood
- Sleep
- Appetite
- Energy levels
- Anhedonia
- Memory
- Concentration
- Motivation
- Guilt
- Self-esteem

Thought Disorder
- Thought alienation
- Thought withdrawal
- Thought broadcast

Passivity
- Somatic passivity

Delusions
- Persecutory delusions
- Paranoid delusions
- Delusions of reference
- Delusions of grandeur
- Delusions of guilt
- Delusions of poverty
- Nihilistic delusions

Fixity and Conviction of Beliefs
- Did these thoughts occur out of the blue or following an unusual experience?
- How convinced are you that you are experiencing this?
- Could there be any other explanation for this?
- Have you told anyone else and what did they say?

Insight
What do you think is happening with you?

Risk Assessment
- Suicidal thoughts or plans
- Deliberate self-harm
- Past psychiatric history
- Substance and alcohol misuse
- Non-compliance with medication [1]

Delusions of Poverty

Scenario

38-year-old Claire Findlater has been referred by the GP after concerns raised by her husband. She has thoughts that she has lost all her money and is now a pauper. The GP has confirmed with her husband, and it is clear that they still have money in their joint bank account.

Task

Perform a mental state examination.

Approach

Hello, I am Dr. _____. I am a psychiatrist. I understand you have been referred by the GP as you are concerned you are now a pauper.

Delusions
- Delusions of poverty—why do you think you have no money anymore?
- Persecutory delusions
- Paranoid delusions
- Delusions of reference
- Delusions of grandeur
- Delusions of guilt
- Nihilistic delusions

Fixity and Conviction of Beliefs
- Did these thoughts occur out of the blue or following an unusual experience?
- How convinced are you that you are experiencing this?
- Could there be any other explanation for this?
- Have you told anyone else and what did they say?

Comment on Appearance and Behaviour

Depression

- Mood
- Sleep
- Appetite
- Energy levels
- Anhedonia
- Memory
- Concentration
- Motivation
- Guilt
- Self-esteem

Thought Disorder

- Thought alienation
- Thought withdrawal
- Thought broadcast

Passivity

- Somatic passivity

Hallucinations

Auditory hallucinations

- How many voices do you hear?
- Do you recognise them?
- Do they talk to you directly?
- Do they talk among themselves about you?
- Do they give you instructions?
- What do they say?
- Do you obey?
- Do they give a running commentary?
- Do you hear the voices in your head or from outside?
- Visual hallucinations

Olfactory hallucinations

Gustatory hallucinations

Tactile hallucinations

Insight

What do you think is happening with you?

Risk Assessment

- Suicidal thoughts or plans
- Deliberate self-harm

- Past psychiatric history
- Substance and alcohol misuse
- Non-compliance with medication [1]

Mania

Scenario

18-year-old Michelle Jones has been referred by the GP as she was behaving in a strange manner. The GP has given her some medication, and she is slightly calmer now.

Task

Perform a mental state examination.

Approach

Hello, I am Dr. _____. I am a psychiatrist. I understand you have been referred by the GP due to some concerns.

- Comment on appearance and behaviour
- Pressured speech

Mania Symptoms
- Mood
- Sleep
- Appetite
- Energy levels
- Concentration
- Self-esteem
- Personal hygiene
- Racing thoughts
- Delusions of grandeur

Insight
What do you think is happening with you?

Risk Assessment
- Reckless driving/speeding
- Overspending

- Special powers like thinking you can fly
- Grand plans/extravagant schemes
- Increased interest in sexual activity
- Substance and alcohol misuse
- Suicidal thoughts or plans
- Deliberate self-harm
- Past psychiatric history [1]

Station-Specific Points

- Please use the time judiciously by interrupting frequently to elicit relevant information.

Delusions of Persecution: Radiation

Scenario

77-year-old Henrietta Reid has been referred by the GP after concerns expressed by her family members. She has informed her family that her neighbours were out to get her.

Task

Perform a mental state examination.

Approach

Hello, I am Dr. _____. I am a psychiatrist. I understand you have been referred by the GP due to some concerns.
   Please tell me more about your difficulties.

Delusions
- Persecutory delusions
- Paranoid delusions
- Delusions of reference
- Delusions of grandeur
- Delusions of guilt
- Delusions of poverty
- Nihilistic delusions

Fixity and Conviction of Beliefs
- Did these thoughts occur out of the blue or following an unusual experience?
- How convinced are you that you are experiencing this?
- Could there be any other explanation for this?
- Have you told anyone else and what did they say?

Comment on Appearance and Behaviour
Depressive Symptoms
- Mood
- Sleep
- Appetite
- Energy levels
- Anhedonia
- Memory
- Concentration
- Motivation
- Guilt
- Self-esteem

Thought Disorder
- Thought alienation
- Thought withdrawal
- Thought broadcast

Passivity
- Somatic passivity

Hallucinations
Auditory hallucinations
  - How many voices do you hear?
  - Do you recognise them?
  - Do they talk to you directly?
  - Do they talk among themselves about you?
  - Do they give you instructions?
  - What do they say?
  - Do you obey them?
  - Do they give a running commentary?
  - Do you hear the voices in your head or from outside?

Visual hallucinations
Olfactory hallucinations
Gustatory hallucinations
Tactile hallucinations

Insight
What do you think is happening with you?

Risk Assessment
- Suicidal thoughts or plans
- Deliberate self-harm
- Past psychiatric history
- Substance and alcohol misuse
- Non-compliance with medication [1]

Delirium Tremens

Scenario

45-year-old Marcus Hyde has been referred by the GP after concerns expressed by his wife that for the last 24 h he had been agitated claiming someone was following him and he could hear them plotting against him. He has a history of alcohol dependence.

Task

Explore psychopathology.

Approach

Hello, I am Dr. _____. I am a psychiatrist. I understand you have been referred by the GP due to some concerns.

History of Alcohol Use
- What do you drink?
- How much do you drink in a day?
- Do you crave for a drink sometimes?
- Do you neglect any other activities that make you happy so you can drink?
- Do you drink first thing in the morning?
- Do you find you have to drink more to achieve the same effect?
- Have you ever tried not to drink?
- What happens when you do not drink—sweating, shakiness, headaches and feeling sick?
- When was the last time you had a drink [2]?

Comment on Appearance and Behaviour
Hallucinations
Auditory hallucinations
- How many voices do you hear?
- Do you recognise them?
- Do they talk to you directly?
- Do they talk among themselves about you?
- Do they give you instructions?
- What do they say?
- Do you obey them?
- Do they give a running commentary?
- Do you hear the voices in your head or from outside?

Visual hallucinations
Olfactory hallucinations
Gustatory hallucinations
Tactile hallucinations

Delusions
- Persecutory delusions
- Paranoid delusions
- Delusions of reference
- Delusions of grandeur

Fixity and Conviction of Beliefs
- Did these thoughts occur out of the blue or following an unusual experience?
- How convinced are you that you are experiencing this?
- Could there be any other explanation for this?
- Have you told anyone else and what did they say?

Depressive Symptoms
- Mood
- Sleep
- Appetite
- Energy levels
- Anhedonia
- Memory
- Concentration

Thought Disorder
- Do you feel someone is interfering with your thoughts?

  Check orientation to time, place and person

Impact
This sounds really difficult for you. How has this impacted on your

- Relationships
- Work—ask about late days and absences

Insight
What do you think is happening with you?

Risk Assessment
- Suicidal thoughts or plans
- Deliberate self-harm
- Past psychiatric history
- Have you ever had fits?
- Driving—driving under the influence of alcohol
- Financial issues
- Health—ulcers, fits, falls and head injury
- Substance misuse [1]

Frontal Lobe Examination

Scenario

75-year-old Benjamin Gault has been having some memory issues with change in personality following a car accident.

Task

Perform a frontal lobe examination.

Approach

Hello, I am Dr. ____. I am a psychiatrist. I would like to perform a few tests to assess your memory.
    May I ask if you have any problems with your hearing or vision?
    I may have to come close to you and touch you to perform some tests.

Orientation to Time, Place and Person
- Time—year, month, season, day of the week and date
- Place—name of this place, floor, city, county and country
- Person—what is your full name, what is your date of birth and how old are you [3, 4]

Lexical Fluency

- In 60 s, please name as many words as possible with the letter 'S' but not names or places.

Similarities

- What is the similarity between a table and a chair?
- What is the similarity between an apple and an orange?

Motor Series

- Luria three-step task—demonstrate the fist, palm and edge three times and each time ask the role player to copy it. Then ask the role player to perform this six consecutive times.

Conflicting Instructions

- When I tap the table twice, may I ask you to tap the table once? When I tap the table once, please tap the table twice.

Go/No-Go Tests

- When I tap the table once, may I ask you to tap the table once? When I tap the table twice, please do not do anything [5].

Abstract Thinking

Cognitive Estimates

- What is the height of an average English gentleman?
- How many camels are there in the UK?

Proverb Interpretation

- What is the meaning of too many cooks spoil the broth?

Alternate Sequencing

Draw an alternate sequence of squares and triangles, and ask the role player to copy the diagram [5, 6].

Cognitive Examination

Scenario

82-year-old Gareth Bissett has been having some memory issues.

Task

Perform a cognitive examination.

Approach

Hello, I am Dr. ___. I am a psychiatrist. I would like to perform a few tests to assess your memory. May I ask if you have any problems with your hearing or vision?

Orientation to Time, Place, and Person
Time—year, month, season, day of the week and date
Place—name of this place, floor, city, county and country
Person—what is your full name, what is your date of birth and how old are you
- Please remember these three words—apple, table and penny. Can you please repeat them? Please remember them and I will ask you later.
- Please spell WORLD. Now please spell it backwards.
- Show two different objects one after the other and ask him to identify them.
- Please repeat this phrase—'No ifs, ands or buts'.
- Please listen to my instructions and perform the following task—take this paper, fold it in half and put it on the table.
- Please repeat the three words that I had requested you to repeat and remember earlier.
- Please write a short sensible sentence that has a subject and verb.
- Please read what I have written here (on the paper write 'please close your eyes') and do what it says.
- Draw intersecting pentagons and ask the role player to copy the diagram.
- Please tell me the name of the prime minister of the UK.
- Please tell me the name of the president of the USA [3, 4].

Cerebellar Examination

Scenario

50-year-old Paula Gilbert has been having some coordination problems.

Task

Perform a cerebellar examination.

Approach

Hello, I am Dr. ___. I am a psychiatrist. I would like to perform a few tests please.

- Check posture.
- Check gait—ataxic gait and broad-based gait.

- Dysarthria—Please say 'west register street'. Please say 'British constitution'. Check for slurred or scanning speech.
- Check for nystagmus.
- Intention tremor—finger-nose test.
- Dysdiadochokinesia.
- Heel-shin test.
- Tandem walking—heel-to-toe walking.
- Romberg's sign.
- Check for hypotonia [7].

References

1. Casey P, Kelly B. Fish's clinical psychopathology signs and symptoms in psychiatry. 3rd ed. The Royal College of Psychiatrists; 2016.
2. Semple D, Smyth R. Assessment of the patient with alcohol problems. Oxford handbook of psychiatry. 3rd ed. Oxford University Press; 2017. p. 552.
3. Zhang M, Ho C, Ho R, Puri B, editors. Get through MRCPsych CASC. Mini mental state assessment. CRC Press Taylor & Francis Group; 2017.
4. Folstein MF, Folstein SE, McHugh PR. "Mini-mental state". A practical method for grading the cognitive state of patients for the clinician. J Psychiatr Res. 1975;12(3):189.
5. Kopp B, Rösser N, Tabeling S, Stürenburg HJ, de Haan B, Karnath HO, et al. Performance on the frontal assessment battery is sensitive to frontal lobe damage in stroke patients. BMC Neurol. 2013;13:13.
6. Zhang M, Ho C, Ho R, Puri B editors. Get through MRCPSych CASC. Frontal lobe assessment. CRC Press Taylor & Francis Group; 2017.
7. Gudlavalleti A, Tenny S. Cerebellar neurological signs. 2021. https://www.ncbi.nlm.nih.gov/books/NBK556080/. Accessed November.

Index

A

Abnormal grief reaction, 19–21
Alcohol dependence, 2, 4, 6, 8, 10, 12, 14, 20,
      63–65, 67, 69, 75, 120
  with anxiety, 68–70
Alcoholic hallucinosis, 70–71
Alcohol use
  complications of, 67–68
  and impact on mood, 74–76
Alzheimer's dementia, 35
Anorexia Nervosa, 93–95
  and mental health act, 96–97
Antidementia, 148–149
Antidepressant induced side
      effects, 17–19
Attention deficit hyperactivity
      disorder, 51–52
Autism spectrum disorder, 49

B

Behavioural and psychological symptoms of
      dementia, 45–46
Bipolar affective disorder, 25
Bodily distress disorder, 82–83
Body dysmorphic disorder, 78–80
Bulimia Nervosa, 91–93

C

Childhood maltreatment, 53–55
Clozapine, 145–146
Cognitive behavioural therapy, 125–126
  for psychosis, 127–129
Cognitive errors, 129
Cognitive examination, 177–178
Complete heart block, 152
Conversion disorder, 77–78

D

Delirium Tremens, 73–74, 174–176
Delusions
  of grandeur, 160–161
  of persecution-radiation, 172–174
  of poverty, 169–171
Dementia, behavioural and psychological
      symptoms of, 45–46
Depression, 28–29
  and myocardial infarction, 26–27
Displacement, 119–121
Dissociative stupor, 85–87
Down's syndrome with dementia,
      55–56
Drug induced psychosis, 114–115

E

Electrocardiogram, 151–153
Electroconvulsive therapy, 146–148
Epilepsy, 13–15
Erotomania, 107–109
Exhibitionism, 101–103
Exposure response prevention, 118–119

F

Family therapy, 124–125
Financial capacity, 157
Fire setting, 110–112
Frontal lobe examination, 176–177
Future violence, 109–110

G

Gender dysphoria, 5–7
Generalised anxiety
      disorder, 7–8

Genetics
    in Alzheimer's disease, 149–150
    of Schizophrenia, 137
GHB dependence, 71–73

H
Hoarding, 158
Hyperprolactinemia, 24–25
Hypochondriasis, 80–82

I
Indecent exposure, 103–105
Interpersonal therapy, 122–124

L
Learning disability and pregnancy, 60–61
Lewy body dementia, 41–43
Lithium, 132–134, 143–145

M
Mania, 43–44, 171–172
Medical capacity, 161
Metabolic syndrome, 15–16
Mild cognitive impairment, 44–45
Morbid jealousy, 105–107
Myocardial infarction, 154

N
Neuroleptic malignant syndrome, 22–23

O
Obsessive compulsive disorder, 3–5
Opiate dependence, 65–66, 138–140
Overdose, 58–59, 84–85

P
Paedophilia, 99–101

Panic disorder, 11–12
Post-partum depression, 136
Post-partum psychosis, 134–136
Post-traumatic stress disorder, 1–3

Q
QTc prolongation, 153

R
Refeeding syndrome, 95–96

S
Schizophrenia, 167–169
    psychosocial treatment for, 126–127
    and substance misuse, 30–31
Self-injurious behaviours, 56
    in learning disability, 56–58
Serotonin syndrome, 16–17
Social anxiety disorder, 9–10
Sodium Valproate, 131, 132
Stalking, 112–113
Systematic desensitisation, 117–118

T
Temporal lobe epilepsy, 13–14
Transference, 121–122
Traumatic brain injury, 87–88
Treatment resistant depression and
        pregnancy, 140–141
Treatment resistant Schizophrenia, 29–30

V
Vascular dementia, 40–41

W
Wandering behaviour, 38–40
Weight gain psychosocial
        chistory, 31–32